# KETO DIET FOR BEGINNERS

## *Burn Fat With The Ketogenic Diet*

by

**Epic Rios**

# Table of Contents

The information in the following pages is broadly considered to be a truthful and accurate account of facts and as such any inattention, use or misuse of the information in question by the reader will render any resulting actions solely under their purview.

There are no scenarios in which the publisher or the original author of this work can be in any fashion deemed liable for any hardship or damages that may befall them after undertaking information described herein.

Additionally, the information in the following pages is intended only for informational purposes and should thus be thought of as universal.

As befitting its nature, it is presented without assurance regarding its prolonged validity or interim quality.

Trademarks that are mentioned are done without written consent and can in no way be considered an endorsement from the trademark holder.

# Introduction

Congratulations on downloading this book and thank you for doing so.

The following chapters will discuss what you need to know to get started on the ketogenic diet.

This diet plan is one of the best diet plans out there because it is effective and it helps you to lose weight and burn off that stubborn fat that you have been working against for a long time.

Simply this effective book will provide you with all of the information that you need to fully understand and follow the ketogenic diet plan.

We will start out with some of the basics of the ketogenic diet, the benefits of this diet plan, how to eat properly, the best meal plans to help you get started, how the ketogenic diet and intermittent fasting can work together, and even how you can modify this diet plan for your workout plan.

Anyone is able to follow the ketogenic diet, and with the help of this educational book, you will be able to see amazing results with your fat and weight loss in no time.

When you have been trying other diet plans for some time and are not seeing the results that you would like, it may be time to change things up and try something new.

The ketogenic diet will effectively help you to see the results that you would like, and this resourceful book will give you all the information that you need to get started.

I want to take the time to thank you so much for choosing this book! Every effort was made to ensure it is full of as much useful information as possible, please enjoy!

# Chapter 1: What is the Ketogenic Diet?

When you are ready to get started on a new diet plan, there are a lot of different options that you can choose from.

Some diets are going to be more like "fasting" where you need to cut out what you eat so much that it is very hard to stick with it. Other diets will focus on cutting out all of the fats that you consume during the day so that you can focus on eating healthy carbs and lots of fruits and vegetables in your diet.

Some diets are healthy and some are not that healthy and there are often many people who swear by these healthy and unhealthy diets. But think about this, which diet is actually going to give you the best results that you would like to practice when it comes to losing weight?

It is important to state that the ketogenic diet is one of the most effective diet plans that you can choose from.

The ketogenic diet plan is simple to understand. In addition, learning and practicing the ketogenic diet is going to take away some of the common misconceptions about dieting, the misconceptions that have been holding you back from losing weight so that you can actually achieve your fat loss goals.

While many traditional diets, the ones that are considered really healthy, will ask you to eat more carbs and cut down on fats, the ketogenic diet takes things in a different direction.

With the ketogenic diet, you are going to severely limit the carbs that you take in and instead replace them with healthy fats that will increase your metabolism and make you feel amazing in no time.

The issue with normal diet plans is that you are taking in too many carbs. These carbs may seem healthy, but when the body breaks them down, they basically become sugars in the body.

If you are consuming additional foods that have sugars in them then this could add some additional issues to your health and prevent you from achieving your weight loss goals.

Keep this in mind - the body is used to consuming carbs for energy. So, the body is very happy when you take in some carbs and the body will use the carbs for energy.

The body will then transfer the carbs over to insulin and then try to use up the insulin. And when the body doesn't use up all of its insulin, then the body simply stores it as fat.

As a result, a person will simply gain weight or not be able to lose fat as a result of the excess insulin.

Unfortunately, carbs are a very effective source of energy for most people. The body will often feel hungry and run down long before you use up the carbs that you consume, and you will eventually feel tired, grumpy, and hungry again. This leads most people to eat more carbs in an effort to get their energy back.

After eating more carbs, people will feel better for a little while. But soon they will be tired and worn out again and the cycle just keeps going on and on.

Eventually you will end up eating way too many calories just to keep your energy levels up and all those extra carbs will be stored as excess body fat.

The ketogenic diet works to break this cycle. Instead of relying so much on eating carbs, you will instead rely on eating healthy fats.

You can still have some carbs, but the point is to push your body into **ketosis, a process where the body will use fats instead of carbs as its main source of energy**.

It is important to state that fat or "healthy fat" can be a really efficient source of energy.

While you will feel worn out and tired for the first few days as the body runs out of carbs (due to you eating fewer carbs), and starts looking for a new energy source, you will soon notice that your energy levels will start to go through the roof.

You will burn the "healthy fat" that you are eating as well as the "fats" that are stored in the body, all while feeling full and satisfied.

When you go on the ketogenic diet, you are responsible for cutting down the number of carbs that you consume.

On the ketogenic diet, most people will be limited to eating no more than fifty grams of carbs each day.  In addition, most of these carbs will come from healthy sources like fruits and vegetables.

Some people like to push themselves into ketosis a little bit faster and will limit themselves to twenty grams of carbs a day or less. However, it is advisable to slowly begin the ketogenic diet and to also slowly begin to reduce the number of carbs you eat each day.

Every person that practices the ketogenic diet needs to experiment with their carb intake based on their activity levels and other factors.

For example, people who do a lot of weightlifting, aerobics and cardio based exercises (swimming, running, etc.,) will need to take in slightly more carbs or above the fifty-gram recommendation to help them stay healthy and so that they can maintain being in ketosis.

**(Ketosis is a process by which the body uses stored fat or body fat as fuel or energy. So, when very little carbs are consumed and that energy is used up, the body will go into ketosis in which the body will look to fat as an energy source for using as fuel or energy.)**

Checking to see if you are in ketosis is very important if you are practicing the ketogenic diet.

You will only lose weight once you reach the state of ketosis and some people may need to adjust their food intake a bit more than others to see some weight loss results.

It is important to state that there are test strips available at pharmacies that you can buy that will allow you to check for the level of ketones in your body, so that you can adjust your diet early on and figure out what changes you need to make to your diet.

**(Ketones are chemical substances that the body produces when there is not enough insulin produced in the body as a result of eating very few carbs. So, the less carbs you eat the less insulin your body will produce resulting in ketones being produced by the body. So, ketones occur as a result of the body using fat as energy or fuel.)**

Remember that when working with the ketogenic diet, you need to change up the way that you are eating on a regular basis.

You are not going to be able to eat a ton of bread and pasta and see results. However, lots of healthy oils and fats from healthy protein sources can help you to get the macronutrients that you need and to lose weight.

Carbs are not completely off limits, but you will be surprised at how quickly your daily allowance will disappear, especially if you are choosing bread and pasta as your carb sources.

Instead, you need to stick with healthy fruits and vegetables and learn how to go with the ones that are lower in carb content compared to others.

This makes it easier to get the vitamins and nutrients that your body needs without pushing the body out of ketosis.

Once you reach ketosis through healthy fats, moderate amounts of protein, and low carbs, you will need to maintain this diet for the long-term.

As soon as you start to eat more carbs and go back to your old habits, you will get out of ketosis and can start to gain the weight again.

You can easily lose a lot of weight with the ketogenic diet, but you need to maintain the ketosis diet for the long-term if you really want to see the good results.

Following the ketogenic diet can be a bit difficult for some people. You may have to give up some of the foods that you have enjoyed in the past.

But once you learn a few of the rules that come with the ketogenic diet and you find a few favorite recipes that will help you to stay within the right macronutrient content for your body and for ketosis you are going to fall in love with the results.

The ketogenic diet may be hard in our modern world, but it is going to give you some amazing results with your weight and fat loss goals.

**Understanding Ketosis**

Ketosis is basically the process of your body relying on fats rather than on carbs or glucose to provide it with energy.

Most people eat enough carbs that they are going to rely on those for their source of energy. But this is not a very efficient form of energy.

You will quickly go through cycles of high energy and then crash when the carbs are all gone, and you will end up eating way more than you need just to keep your energy levels up.

With ketosis, you do not need to worry about your energy levels crashing and then trying to eat more carbs in order to increase your energy levels again.  Instead, you will teach the body to stop relying on carbs and instead the body will learn to rely on healthy fats that you start to take in.

When you eat healthy fats, ketones are going to be produced and used for energy. Ketones will replace the glucose, giving you plenty of healthy energy without having to worry about the horrible crashes that glucose (sugars from carbs) causes.

**Eating on the Ketogenic Diet**

When you follow a ketogenic diet, you will consume at least 70 percent of your calories each day from fat. The majority of the rest will come from protein, with only about five percent coming from healthy sources of carbs, such as low-carb vegetables.

As a beginner, you will need to build your meals around healthy sources of fats. These can include oils, cheese, nuts, meats, and fatty fish. You can then add in some healthy sources of protein if they are not included already, as well as healthy low-carb options like vegetables and some fruits.

One thing to keep in mind on this diet plan is that you still need to take in moderate amounts of protein.

Many people get so focused on the fat intake and limiting their carbs that they forget to take in enough protein. Protein is important to help you stay full and for preserving your body's muscles as well as keeping your muscles strong.

**Negative Effects of This Diet Plan**

You may also wonder if there are any negative effects of following this diet plan.

Plain and simple, you are taking a large food group (carbs) and cutting it down to almost nothing on this diet plan.

For the most part, as soon as your body has time to adapt to ketosis, there shouldn't be any negative effects that you need to deal with.

You may feel a bit tired in the beginning as your body adapts, but once that adaption happens, you will find that you have more energy than ever before.

You should make sure that you have a wide variety of food options when it comes to eating on the ketogenic diet plan.

If you eat the same meals each day, or the same vegetables, you are going to miss out on important nutrients and this can cause some negative effects. This is true of any diet plan if you do not add in variety.

Make sure that you get plenty of variety in the diet, and you will see amazing results without any negative side effects.

**Do I Need to Measure Ketones?**
Many people choose to monitor the ketones that they consume. Actually, it is important that you monitor your ketones in order to ensure that you reach ketosis and that you stay within it to see weight loss results.

It is not necessarily a requirement for the diet plan, but it certainly helps. Measuring your ketones does not have to be difficult.

There are some testing strips that you can use that will tell you when you have entered ketosis and you can bring these out any time that you are worried about whether you are in the right range with your carbs or not.

**Who Uses the Ketogenic Diet?**
The biggest reason that people will choose to go on the ketogenic diet is to simply lose weight.

When you start relying on fat for your source of energy rather than glucose (sugars), you can melt off the weight and fat in no time. However, there are many other reasons that people may choose to practice the ketogenic diet.

Originally, the ketogenic diet was designed to help patients who were dealing with a variety of neurological conditions, especially epilepsy. It was found that young children who relied on a ketogenic-like diet were able to reduce the frequency of their seizures and reduce their medications.

Believe it or not, but there are some athletes who like to use the ketogenic diet to help with their endurance.

According to a paper that was released in the European Journal of Clinical Nutrition, there are a few other reasons that someone may choose to use the ketogenic diet. These include:

- Evidence that the ketogenic diet can help people with high cholesterol, type 2 diabetes, weight loss, and epilepsy.

- New evidence has shown how the ketogenic diet may be able to help with a variety of neurological diseases like brain trauma, narcolepsy, Alzheimer's, and Parkinson's Disease, to name a few.

- People that suffer from cancer, severe acne, and even polycystic ovarian syndrome are often helped with the ketogenic diet as well.

Basically, anyone is able to use the ketogenic diet, whether they want to lose weight or are working to avoid one of the conditions named above. The ketogenic diet is easy to follow and gives such amazing benefits to those who are able to follow it.

# Chapter 2: The Benefits of the Ketogenic Diet

There are a lot of reasons that people will choose to use and practice the ketogenic diet.

Simply, the ketogenic diet is one of the most effective diet plans out there. In addition, the ketogenic diet can help resolve a variety of health issues that people are dealing with and not just with weight loss.

Some of the great benefits that you will receive when you decide to use and practice the ketogenic diet are:

- **Lose weight:** The number one reason that people choose to use the ketogenic diet is that they want to lose weight. And this diet plan is very effective at helping this to happen.

   Once your body enters into the process of ketosis and starts relying on fats for energy rather than carbs, you will see the weight melt off in no time.

- **Next, the ketogenic diet can help reduce cancer:** Some studies have shown how the ketogenic diet may be effective at reducing your risks of developing cancer.

Cancer cells thrive when given lots of carbs, so if you take these carbs away, they will basically starve out. Regular healthy cells can rely on healthy fats for their nutrition, but cancer cells can't.

- **Next, the ketogenic diet will give you more energy:** During the first few days on the ketogenic diet, you may notice that you are feeling tired and worn down. This is because the body is so used to relying on carbs to stay energetic.

When you take those carbs away, the body is not sure where to find its energy source and may feel run down. You just need to give it a few days, though; the body will start using the fats that you provide it for energy in no time. Once that happens, you will have more energy than ever before.

- **Next, the ketogenic diet will help lower your risk of diabetes:** With all those carbs you traditionally eat, it is common to see a risk of diabetes.

You have to be very careful of the carbs you eat because the body will treat some carbs you eat just like sugars once they are eaten and broken down.

So, if you are eating some sugars and lots of carbs, you are raising your insulin levels and increasing the amount of risk you have for diabetes.

Cut out a lot of those carbs, as well as the sugars, and your body can clean itself up and cut down on your risk of diabetes.

- **Next, the ketogenic diet will lower your blood pressure:** Many people who have gone on the ketogenic diet report that their blood pressures went down.

Many of the foods that you consume on a regular diet will have a ton of sodium inside, which can raise your blood pressure. Add in all the processed foods, high amount of carbs, and even the bad fats, and it is no wonder that most people have bad high blood pressure.

The ketogenic diet cuts out a lot of these bad unhealthy foods out of your diet so that you can recover and get that blood pressure back to normal.

- **Next, the ketogenic diet is great for the heart:** The ketogenic diet can even help out with the health of your heart.

  The healthy fats that you consume will help to strengthen your heart. The healthy fats also deliver some of those healthy vitamins and nutrients over to the heart better than carbs do.

  So, once you are reducing some of the carbs, the ones that turn into sugars in the body, you are giving the heart a fighting chance to be healthy and strong again.

- **Next, the ketogenic diet clears the mind:** When you are able to cut down on the number of carbs that you consume, and the number of calories that you are consuming, you will find that your mind feels much clearer.

  It will feel amazing to remember things, to think things through critically, and to no longer have to deal with the brain fog that you may have suffered from before as a result of eating so many carbs.

- **Next, the ketogenic diet can help fight epilepsy:** Originally, the ketogenic diet was developed as a way to help children who were suffering from chronic epilepsy.

The high fat and low carb ketogenic diet were effective at helping young children fight off epilepsy and kept the episodes away.

The ketogenic diet needed to be used over the long-term, usually for two years or more, but helped children to not have to deal with the horrible effects of their seizures and helped them to reduce the amount of medication they needed to take.

Almost everyone is able to benefit from the use of the ketogenic diet. It is different compared to some of the other diet plans that are available on the market, but this is part of what makes it so successful compared to the other diet plans.

When you are ready to start losing weight and improving many other aspects of your health, then make sure to try out the ketogenic diet to help you out.

# Chapter 3: The Side Effects of the Ketogenic Diet

Before you get started with the ketogenic diet, it is important to know that there are some side effects or using and practicing the ketogenic diet.

These side effects are not horrible side effects like what you may be used to with common medications, but it is still a good idea to know what to expect when you are getting started on this new diet plan.

Some of the side effects that you may encounter when you are on the ketogenic diet are:

**Dizziness or Headaches**

One of the first side effects that you may experience when you get started with the ketogenic diet includes dizziness and headaches.

Dizziness and headaches are really prevalent in those individuals who for a very long time consumed a lot of caffeine and sugar before starting the ketogenic diet.

Both caffeine and sugar are highly addictive and if you go cold turkey on them, you may have a few side effects during the beginning process of the ketogenic diet.

You may introduce a little caffeine or sugar later on in the ketogenic diet plan if you want, but for those individuals who experience having a lot of trouble starting this diet plan or who really are addicted to caffeine and sugar, it is best to cut them out completely.

The good news is that the symptoms of withdrawal are only going to last for a few days and they really are not that severe.

You may feel a little anxious or upset because you will crave the caffeine and sugars that you are trying to eliminate from your diet.

However, if you are able to overcome your cravings for caffeine and sugar during the initial process of the ketogenic diet, you will break the addictions and you will not feel so reliant on consuming them as much.

One thing that you may decide to try is to slowly cut out your sugar and caffeine intake before you go on the ketogenic diet. This will help you to not have to deal with these withdrawal symptoms as much. This can make things easier since you will already be dealing with feeling tired as your body gets used to the fats instead of the carbs.

If you are thinking about going on the ketogenic diet, consider cutting down on the sugars and caffeine for at least a few weeks ahead of time and you will not have to deal with the headaches or the dizziness as much when you begin.

**Leg Cramps**

Some of those who decide to go on the ketogenic diet will complain of dealing with leg cramps, especially when they are trying to go to bed at night.

This is common when you are in the early phase of the ketogenic diet. This is a big problem for those users who are not paying attention to their micronutrients on this diet plan and who are not taking in enough potassium on this diet plan.

There are a few things that you are able to do to make sure you are getting enough potassium.

You can first work to try and eat plenty of foods with healthy amounts of potassium in them. If you are having trouble doing this, you may decide to take a supplement that has potassium inside of it.

Many beginners decide to take a potassium supplement to help prevent leg cramps because keeping track of the macronutrients and the micronutrients for good health can be difficult.

However, you need to work towards not depending on supplements and instead eat real foods that will provide you with all the nutrients your body needs without taking any supplements.

## Constipation

If you are not watching your micronutrients when you are on the ketogenic diet, you may deal with the issue of constipation. This can be really uncomfortable for most people to deal with and can make sticking with the ketogenic diet a bit difficult. However, the solution to this problem is pretty simple.

To ensure that you are not going to deal with constipation on the ketogenic diet plan, make sure that the majority of carbs that you decide to eat come from healthy green vegetables, which are full of fiber.

You also need to drink a lot of water on this diet plan because water has been shown to combat and prevent constipation. For those individuals who maybe are already dealing with constipation, you may try a laxative to help you out.

## Bad Breath

Another side effect that you may need to deal with on the ketogenic diet is bad breath.

While on the ketogenic diet plan, the body is going to burn up fat so that you can use this fat as energy. This is the process of ketosis and will help you to burn through fat in your diet and the fat that is sitting around your body.

Unfortunately, the ketones (burning fat used as energy) that are released in this process will leave you with bad breath and make your urine smell bad.

The smell is going to be a little bit different than you may experience when after eating smelly food or by those individuals who suffer from halitosis (bad breath resulting from health problems).

Some people even compare it to a fruity candy smell instead, but if you do not want your breath to smell at all, then it is important to find a few ways to get rid of the bad breath.

Chewing on some gum without sugar, using mouthwash, or chewing on parsley or mint can help to get rid of this smell while keeping you on the ketogenic diet.

**Feeling Tired**

There are many people who will get started on the ketogenic diet who claim they feel tired.

They get going on this plan and are excited about all the big promises of more energy when they eat more healthy fats and fewer carbs.

Then they start on this diet and the first few days or in the first week they will begin to feel really tired almost like they just don't have enough energy to get things done.

This is completely normal on the ketogenic diet and it is important to know that these energy lacking feelings are going to fade away pretty soon.

The reason that you feel so tired when you start the ketogenic diet is that the body basically doesn't have any fuel for energy.

Sure, you are taking in healthy foods and providing it with fuel, but the body is used to relying on carbs and doesn't know what it should do when you take the majority of those carbs away.

So, the body is basically searching around hoping that you will eat and take in the carbs that it needs for easy energy access. When you don't eat carbs or consume enough carbs your body is basically working on very little to no energy for a little while.

The good news is that feeling tired is not going to last for a very long time. For most people, it takes less than a week for the body to start recognizing the fat as a good source of energy and it will switch over.

Once the body starts to realize that it can use fat for energy instead of carbs, you will start to notice a big change. Your energy will come back in a big way and you will feel amazing in no time. You will be able to keep going all day long, even with fewer calories, and will ensure that you feel great about this diet plan.

As you can see, none of these side effects are life-threatening or that big of a deal when it comes to the ketogenic diet.

These side effects can make you a little bit uncomfortable and may not be the most pleasant when you are dealing with bad breath and feeling tired.

However, these side effects will usually not last for a long time and once your body adjusts to the ketogenic diet plan, you will not have to worry about them any longer.

# Chapter 4: Who Can Safely Go on the Ketogenic Diet?

In most cases, following the ketogenic diet is a great experience.

There are so many great health benefits that you will be able to enjoy when it comes to the ketogenic diet.

Many people choose to go on the ketogenic diet because they are tired of not being able to lose weight or fight off all that excess fat that has been hanging around their body for a long time.

But weight loss is not the only reason that you may choose to go on the ketogenic diet. If you have been fighting diabetes and its side effects for some time, reducing the number of carbs and the glucose it produces can help combat this health issue.

If you are worried about your high cholesterol levels and high blood pressure, simply practicing and following the ketogenic diet plan can help you to reduce your risks with these health issues as well.

Even younger children who have been dealing with epilepsy and those children with other neurological conditions may be able to benefit with the help of the ketogenic diet.

The children may be able to reduce some of the symptoms that they are dealing with and some have even been able to no longer need to use the medication they are on when they accurately follow the ketogenic diet plan.

Anyone who is dealing with health diseases or wants to lose weight or just simply wants to live a healthier lifestyle will be able to discover that the ketogenic diet is a good tool to help them out.

It doesn't matter if you are a man or a woman, the ketogenic diet is the right option to help anyone.

**Who Shouldn't Use the Ketogenic Diet?**
There are so many people who are able to use the ketogenic diet. The ketogenic diet has a lot of benefits and it can help you to lose weight, fight off many health concerns, and help you to feel amazing in no time.

However, there are certain groups of people who should avoid and not practice the ketogenic diet.

Practicing the ketogenic diet plan can be detrimental to the health of some people and even make them feel sick. Some of those individuals who should avoid the ketogenic diet are:

- Children and teenagers
- Women who are pregnant and breastfeeding
- Women with irregular menstrual cycles
- People that have issues with their thyroid glands
- People that suffer from adrenal fatigue
- High-level athletes who need carbs to help them function better

These groups of people will often not do as well with the ketogenic diet. This is because they need special dietary requirements that are eliminated from their diet when they follow the ketogenic diet.

For example, a pregnant or nursing mother needs to take in carbs to help her baby to grow and eliminating these completely can result in a nutrient deficiency for the baby.

Teenagers and children often need some of the glucose that is found in carbs, or they need higher carb content from fruits and vegetables than the ketogenic diet allows.

This does not mean that these groups of people can't take some advice from the ketogenic diet to help them stay healthy.

For example, teenagers or pregnant women may choose to limit their carbs a bit, but not to the fifty grams a day that is recommended by the ketogenic diet.

Instead, teenagers or pregnant women can instead stick to eating healthy carbs like fruits and vegetables while reducing their intake of unhealthy carbs like the bread and pastas that they normally eat.

Teenagers or pregnant women can also consider increasing their healthy fat intake and eating good amounts of protein each day.

So basically, some of these groups of people can follow some of the principles of the ketogenic diet without following or practicing so many of the restrictions the actual diet requires.

If you fall into one of the groups above, it may be a good idea to talk to your doctor before attempting to go on this diet plan.

This will help you to determine if you really need the ketogenic diet and if it is actually a healthy option for you, especially if you are in one of the groups above.

# Chapter 5: The Ketogenic Diet and Exercise

It is important to understand how exercise and your fitness performance can be affected by the ketogenic diet.

It is also important to understand that maybe your exercise routine/plan/goals may need to be changed a little bit as a result of practicing the ketogenic diet.

However, you will still see some great results from your fitness workouts while practicing the ketogenic diet. In additional, habitual exercise combined with the ketogenic diet will help you to lose weight and fat faster than ever.

You may also need to add a few extra carbs to your diet in order to have the right amount of energy for achieving your health and fitness goals.

With the ketogenic diet, you are greatly reducing the number of carbs that you are consuming and since many athletes require carbs to help them stay energetic, you may be curious to know how this is going to affect your body when you enter ketosis.

You will need to keep a few things in mind when you get started on the ketogenic diet when it comes to exercising, but it is just fine to exercise on this diet and all the health benefits definitely make it worth your time.

First, we need to understand that the traditional view on weight loss, the idea that you just need to eat less and exercise for a longer period of time (while getting plenty of cardio in as well) is advice that is outdated and just won't work with the ketogenic diet.

To really lose weight and get that leaner frame that you have been looking for, the foods that you eat while on the ketogenic diet are what matter the most.

Eating recommended foods on the ketogenic diet like meats, seafood, and dairy are great ways to begin the ketogenic diet.

The most important thing you can do for weight loss and maintaining your energy levels is to pay attention to how well and how disciplined you are to following the ketogenic diet.

If you are able to remain in a steady state of ketosis, rather than coming in and out of it because you can't keep your carbs steady or low, you will see some amazing results.

Before you decide to start doing more and more of your regular physical exercise activities while on the ketogenic diet, make sure that you understand when your body is in ketosis as well as spend some time testing your ketone levels.

However, once you get used to how the ketogenic diet works, adding in exercise can provide you with a lot of good benefits to your health.

Physical exercise like strength training and lifting weights will help to make your bones stronger as well as build muscle and make you have that lean look you want.

In addition, physical exercise like strength training and lifting weights is also great for the heart. And as long as you are taking in nutrients properly on the ketogenic diet, physical exercise can easily fit in with your new diet plan.

Just remember that when you are exercising while on the ketogenic diet, make sure to stay healthy, make sure your energy levels are good and don't harm yourself while practicing the ketogenic diet.

**Why Should I Exercise on the Ketogenic Diet?**

After learning a bit more about ketosis and how the body needs higher levels of carbs in order to properly perform the activities that you would like, you may think that ketosis is not the best for long-term exercise.

However, exercising while on the ketogenic diet actually provides the user with many benefits including:

- In one study, ultra-endurance athletes were asked to do a three-hour run. Those who ate a low carb diet for about twenty months on average had up to three times the fat burn compared to the athletes who followed a high-carb diet. Both of these groups were able to replenish the same amount of muscle glycogen when done.

- Studies have shown that ketosis can help to prevent fatigue in people who exercise for long periods of time.

  For example, people that strength train for 1 or 2 hours or people who do cardio exercise activities such as running have sufficient energy to complete their long workouts.

- Ketosis is great for helping to maintain your blood glucose levels, whether you are considered obese or not.

- With the help of keto-adaption (which we will talk about later on), low-carb ketogenic dieters are actually better able to perform various activities, even while taking in fewer carbs over time.

- You receive all the regular benefits of exercise. In addition to the benefits listed above, those individuals who are on the ketogenic diet are able to receive all the same benefits that they would receive on any other diet while working out.

  However, the main difference between the ketogenic diet and other diets is that the ketogenic diet uses fat as energy instead of carbs.

  Keep this in mind, exercising while on the ketogenic diet will help you to be in a better mood, lose weight, see fat loss, control your blood sugar levels, reduce blood pressure, and so much more.

Everyone should consider starting on their own workout program and combining it with the ketogenic diet.

It is important to state that having a good mixture of different exercises, from flexibility to strength training and some lower-intensity aerobics or cardio exercises, will help you to make the whole body strong and will prevent injuries along the way.

While you may need to take a little bit of time off from working out when you first get started with the ketogenic diet to help you adjust, most people are able to successfully work out while practicing the ketogenic diet.

By making a few adjustments to your ketogenic lifestyle and by watching how many carbs you eat as well as when you consume your carbs will make all the difference in the results that you see when it comes to achieving your weight loss goals.

**Types of Exercises to do While on the Ketogenic Diet**
Your nutritional needs are going to vary based on the exercise or exercises that you want to perform. But generally, you will be able to divide up exercises into four group.

These four groups of exercises include stability training, flexibility training, anaerobic exercises, and aerobic exercises. Let's take a look at how each of these can work with the ketogenic diet:

- **Aerobic exercise:** Aerobic exercise is typically known as cardio (swimming, running, cycling) and it will be any activity that gets the heart up and running for more than three minutes. As a result, your body may require more carbs while practicing the ketogenic diet.

If you do cardio exercises that are steady-state and lower in intensity like walking you are going to be concentrating on fat burning, which makes it a great exercise for the ketogenic diet.

- **Anaerobic exercise:** This type of exercise is going to have short bursts of energy throughout an exercise session, such as HIIT, powerlifting or explosive exercises.

  If you plan to do anaerobic exercises, you may need to take in more carbs because anaerobic exercises require a lot more carbs as their primary fuel source.

  Make sure that when you combine anaerobic exercises with the ketogenic diet that you consume just a little more carbs just for the sake of making sure you have the necessary energy to complete your physical workouts.

- **Flexibility training:** It is a good idea to add some flexibility exercises to your fitness routine.

  Flexibility training can be helpful for stretching out the muscles, improving your range of motion, and supporting the joints.

Flexibility training is often used to help prevent injuries from some of the other workouts that you may do.

Some examples of flexibility training are Yoga and just simple stretching exercises. Flexibility training does not require a lot of carbs. As a result, the ketogenic diet is perfect for people that do Yoga or simple stretching exercises.

- **Stability exercises:** Stability exercises are exercises that work on your core or abdominal (abs) muscles as well as help improve your balance.

Stability exercises are good for helping control your body's movements, strengthen the muscles in the body, and can even improve your body's alignment. Stability exercises do not require a lot of carbs.

As a result, the ketogenic diet is perfect for people that practice stability exercises.

Keep this in mind when you are exercising while practicing the ketogenic diet:

**Mix up your workouts as much as possible.**

**Do a combination of all four types of exercises and or training mentioned above for the purpose of developing the type of body that you want.**

**At the same time always monitor your energy levels to make sure you are consuming just enough carbs while practicing the ketogenic diet.**

**If at any moment you are feeling too tired to complete your workout routine simply stop exercising, monitor your energy levels and see if you need to increase your carbs intake. Always think safety first.**

It is important to state that as you practice the ketogenic diet and you reach ketosis, the intensity of your exercise workouts is going to matter quite a bit.

When you do low-intensity workouts like walking or Yoga, the body will rely more on fat as its energy source, so these workouts are the best for those on the ketogenic diet.

The high-intensity aerobic exercises, like jogging and running, and anaerobic exercises, like powerlifting and sprinting, are going to rely more on carbs as an energy source and are not the best exercises to do while practicing the ketogenic diet.

Just keep in mind that if you are going to do high-intensity exercises you may need to add some more carbs to your diet.


**Picking a Targeted Ketogenic Diet (Variations)**

So far, we have just been talking about the basic ketogenic diet. This is a great diet if you are looking to get started and you don't plan to do really intense workouts.

The ketogenic diet will often work for regular exercise and for a little bit of low-intensity activities as well.

But if you are planning on doing activities that are more intense, or you plan to exercise or workout more than three days out of the week to help with weight and fat loss, then it is time to consider a targeted ketogenic diet variation.

A targeted ketogenic diet variation will help you to adjust your diet so that you get enough carbs to help you achieve your fitness goals as well as keep you in ketosis.

Those higher intensity workouts, like lots of weightlifting and sprinting are not going to do well with the regular ketogenic diet so having a targeted ketogenic diet variation will help you get the results that you would like.

These targeted ketogenic diet variations will allow you to have some more carbs during the day so that you can maintain your activity levels. This does not mean that you can go out and enjoy as many sodas and baked goods as you like.

You still need to get your carbs from keto approved foods, like fruits and vegetables, but you are allowed to increase your healthy carb intake.

A good thing to remember is that you should eat about 15 to 30 grams of fast acting carbs (which includes options like fruit) about twenty minutes before and after your workout.

This helps your muscles to get the glycogen that they need to do well during training and so that your muscles can recover.

Eating during that time period will ensure that the carbs are used for the workout, so you won't leave ketosis at all.

**Options or Variations of the Ketogenic Diet**

There are a few options for the ketogenic diet that you can pick based on the amount of physical activity that you plan to do. The different ketogenic diet variations that you can choose from include:

- **The standard ketogenic diet:** With this diet option you will keep your total carb count between 20 to 50 grams each day.

- **The targeted ketogenic diet:** With this diet option, you will stick with the 20 to 50 grams of carbs each day. But you will plan out when you eat these carbs. You will want to get the majority, if not all, of these carbs about an hour or less before you do your exercise.

  This is the best option for athletes who like to do high-intensity activities like weightlifting, sprinting, CrossFit, etc.,

- **The cyclical ketogenic diet:** For this one, you will cut your carbs down to almost nothing for a few days. And then on the days that you want to do a higher-intensity workout, you will eat higher-carbs on that day. This should even out for the right amount of carbs throughout the week.

Depending on the exercises that you are doing you may find that the carb content is too low, and you are not taking in enough carbs to keep up with your activity levels.

If you want to know if you are in a state of ketosis, you can simply purchase some test strips at the local pharmacy that will help you to know whether you are in ketosis or not.

You may also be able to increase your carb intake a little bit and still remain in the state of ketosis.

However, it is important to be careful when you slightly increase your carbs intake because it is really easy to jump out of ketosis.

In addition, if you do jump out of ketosis then you will lose the benefits of the ketogenic diet plan if you aren't closely monitoring how many carbs you consume.

The good news is that most people are able to adapt to eating lower-carb diets and using fat to help them get the fuel that they need.

This may take a few weeks and you may not be as strong for those first few weeks as the body adjusts.

However, the longer you remain on the ketogenic diet, the more the body can adapt to this diet plan.

After practicing the ketogenic diet for a while, your body will become more efficient at burning the fat and using up the ketones that are in the body.

With enough physical exercise and after a while of being on the ketogenic diet, you will be able to see some amazing results with your body as well as achieve whatever fitness goals you plan to achieve.

# Chapter 6: What Should I Eat on the Ketogenic Diet?

One question that a lot of people will ask when getting started on the ketogenic diet is what they are allowed to eat.

Working with the right macronutrients is one of the most important parts of the ketogenic diet.

You must make sure that you are eating plenty of healthy fats and low carbs so that you can stay in ketosis.

Actually, eating plenty of healthy fats and low carbs is going to be one of the most important things that you concentrate on when it comes to the ketogenic diet.

However, as long as the foods that you eat fit into these macronutrients, and you are getting plenty of vitamins and minerals from the fruits and vegetables you choose to eat, you will lose weight.

Before we look at the specific foods that you are able to eat on the ketogenic diet let's take a look at the macronutrients.

This is really important and will ensure that you are eating enough fats to stay energetic as well as keeping the carbs low enough so that you don't kick yourself out of ketosis.
Also, don't forget that it is important to eat healthy sources of protein rich foods so that you can keep your muscles big and strong.

First, let's take a look at the fats that you need to eat. It is recommended that you get somewhere between 70 to 75 percent of your daily calories from healthy fats.

You must make sure that these are healthy fats.

Going to the local fast food restaurant and eating a big burger and fries will not count because these are bad fats that will not help out with the ketogenic diet. Instead, eating healthy fats like olive oil, fats from dairy products, and fats that come in healthy protein sources are much better options.

You will also need to eat moderate amounts of protein as well. You will need between 15 and 20 percent of your daily calories from protein.

This helps to keep the muscles as strong as possible and can be especially important if you are someone who likes to work out a lot and wants to build muscle with the ketogenic diet plan. Stick with options like healthy fish, chicken, turkey, and ground beef.

And finally, most people will want to keep their carb intake down to five percent or lower.

However, if you are really into weight lifting, you can sometimes go up to ten percent. But, before you increase your carbs intake, make sure that you experiment and see if you are really in ketosis with the higher amount of carbs.

Remember, when choosing carbs to eat stick with healthy options like fruits and vegetables that will help to keep you feeling full. In addition, eating healthy carbs like fruits and vegetables will give your body the vitamins and nutrients that your body needs.

If you are able to stick with these macronutrients, you will see great results with the ketogenic diet. It will take some time to get used to which foods will fit into this diet plan, but once you get used to it, losing weight and fat will be easier than ever before.

**Foods to Eat on the Ketogenic Diet**
Sticking with the macronutrients that we talked about above is one of the most important things that you can do on this diet plan.

But putting this into a meal plan can be difficult when you first get started. Some of the foods that you are able to enjoy when following the ketogenic diet include:

- **Meat:** There are many different types of meat that you can enjoy, and this will provide you with the protein and some of the fats that you need.

  You can choose from options like fish, lamb, veal, pork, venison, chicken, quail, duck, and shellfish. With chicken, make sure that you leave the skin on to help increase the fat content, but do not bread or batter any poultry that you eat.

  Make sure that you do not eat any processed meats, though. If choosing canned fish options, make sure that the preservation method does not use any added sugar.

- **Eggs:** Many meals on the ketogenic diet will require you to eat eggs for the purpose of consuming both protein and healthy fat. Because eggs have lots of healthy protein and fats, they can be eaten for breakfast, lunch or dinner.

- **Cheese:** For the most part, cheese is a good food to eat while on the ketogenic diet.

There are a few carbs found in the different varieties of cheese, so make sure to read the labels carefully and then count the carbs before you eat them.

Some cheese may push you over your daily required carbs intake so make sure you keep track of other carbs you have eaten that day.

- **Vegetables:** Vegetables will contain most of the carbs that you are going to eat, but try to keep this to a minimum.

You should go with the green and leafy options because these are lower in carbs so options like lettuce, cabbage, kale, and watercress are great.

You can also go with options like bean sprouts, cucumber, celery, broccoli, and asparagus.

- **Fruits:** You can enjoy some fruits on the ketogenic diet, but you need to be careful about which ones you eat.

Some fruits can be higher in carbs compared to some of the other food options on the list and if you eat too many fruits, you will end up going over your daily required carbs intake.

If you choose to add some fruits to your diet, carefully watch your portions and avoid going over on the carb content.

One recommended fruit is the avocado. The avocado is a good source of healthy fat so try to make the avocado part of your ketogenic diet meal plan.

- **Nuts:** Nuts are a good source of healthy fats and protein so they are fine to eat as long as you eat them in moderation as a type of dessert or as a snack. Some recommended nuts are walnuts.

- **Cream, butter, and oils** are usually fine because they provide you with some healthy sources of fat.

- **Dry spices** and **fresh herbs** are great for the ketogenic diet. Dry spices and fresh herbs will help you to get some flavoring in your meals without adding in any extra carbs.

As you can see, while you do need to be careful with the macronutrients that you are consuming on the ketogenic diet, there are still some options that you can go with to eat great meals.

Mix and match some of the options that were mentioned above, and you will get tasty meals that are easy to make and will help you to lose weight without feeling hungry.

**Foods to Avoid on the Ketogenic Diet**

For the most part, if the foods are not listed in the section above, you should not consume them on the ketogenic diet.

Consuming foods that are not recommended for the ketogenic diet can add in too many bad fats, bad carbs, and sugars than your body does not need. In addition, consuming foods that are not recommended for the ketogenic diet may kick you out of your ketosis state.

Keep in mind that you do not want to work hard to get into ketosis and then end up cheating yourself and getting kicked out of ketosis because you consumed foods that are not recommended for the ketogenic diet.

Some of the foods that you will need to avoid on the ketogenic diet are:

- **Bread and pasta:** Bread and pasta may seem healthy, but just a small serving can put you over your required daily carb intake.

  There are healthier alternatives, such as keto bread or using vegetables to make noodles, so you can still enjoy some of your favorite meals without having to worry about eating too many carbs.

- **Baked goods:** In between the excess carbs and sugars that are inside most baked goods, it is no wonder that baked goods are not allowed on the ketogenic diet.

  It is best to stick with eating a piece of fruit (especially if you can find one that is lower in carbs) for your snack rather than eating any of the baked goods that are available.

- **Processed frozen foods/meals:** Anything that you can find in the freezer section of your grocery store should be avoided.

  These frozen foods may seem healthy, but the preservatives and carbs are extremely high and will kick you out of ketosis.

  It is best to just leave everything that is in the freezer section alone and stick with fresh and whole foods instead.

- **Sodas:** Some people choose to drink diet sodas when they are on the ketogenic and diet sodas are allowed. However, you should avoid regular sodas because of all the sugar that is inside of them.

- **Fast foods:** While you are on the ketogenic diet, you need to avoid going out to eat.

  Fast foods are full of way too many carbs and bad fats and will instantly take you out of ketosis without much effort.

  Avoid fast foods and just cook your meals at home instead.

- **Deli meats:** Deli meats may seem like a good option to get your protein, but in reality, they are mostly processed and full of lots of carbs.

  It is best to avoid deli meats as much as possible and focus your time and energy on eating healthier proteins and carbs.

It is important that you eat the right foods when it comes to the ketogenic diet.

There are some other diet plans that will allow you to cheat on occasion, but when you cheat on the ketogenic diet, you lose all of your weight loss benefits.

If you would like to stay in ketosis and really lose weight, then make sure to avoid the foods mentioned above and you will see great results with the ketogenic diet.

# Chapter 7: Simple Meal Plans for the Ketogenic Diet

One of the hardest things that many beginners have trouble with is figuring out what they need to eat on the ketogenic diet.

While they may understand how the macronutrients are supposed to work on the diet, they are worried about how to plan out their meals and how to make it work well for them.

Coming up with ideas for your ketogenic meal plans is one of the best things that you can do because it outlines what you need to eat for the whole week or longer if you like.

Now, we are going to look at a simple one-week meal plan that you can follow to get started on the ketogenic diet and see amazing results in no time.

**Monday**

Breakfast:  Scrambled Eggs

Lunch:      Keto Asian Salad

Dinner:     Pesto Chicken Casserole

**Tuesday**

Breakfast:     Cheese Roll-ups

Lunch:          Caprese Omelet

Dinner:          Meat Pie

**Wednesday**

Breakfast:     Frittata with Spinach

Lunch:          Chicken Soup (No Noodle)

Dinner:          Carbonara

**Thursday**

Breakfast:     Dairy Free Latte

Lunch:          Avocado and Goat Cheese Salad

Dinner:          Keto Pizza

**Friday**

Breakfast:     Mushroom Omelet

Lunch:          Smoked Salmon

Dinner:          Keto Tacos

**Saturday**

Breakfast:     Baked Bacon Omelet

Lunch:          Keto Quesadillas

Dinner:          Asian Stir-Fry

**Sunday**

Breakfast:    Berry Pancakes

Lunch:        Italian Keto Plate

Dinner:       Pork Chops

**Keto Recipes**

**Recipe #1**

***Scrambled Eggs***

What's in it?

- Some salt

- Pepper

- Butter (1 oz.)

- Eggs (2)

**How's it done?**

1. Whisk together the eggs while adding the pepper and salt.

2. Add some butter to a skillet and let it warm up. When the butter is hot, pour the eggs and let them cook.

3. After two minutes, the eggs should be creamy, and you can finish scrambling and enjoy!

**Keto Recipe #2**

*Pesto Chicken Casserole*

What's in it?

- Peppers
- Some salt
- Chopped garlic cloves (1)
- Diced feta cheese (8 oz.)
- Pitted olives (8 Tbsp.)
- Heavy whip cream (1.5 cups)
- Green pesto (3 oz.)
- Butter (2 oz.)
- Chicken thighs (1.5 lbs.)
- Leafy greens (5.3 oz.)
- Olive oil (4 Tbsp.)

**How's it done?**

1. Allow the oven to heat up to 400 degrees. While the oven is heating up, cut up the chicken thighs into pieces and season them with pepper and salt.

2. Add the chicken to a skillet and fry them with some butter to make them nice and brown.

3. In another bowl, mix together the heavy cream and the pesto. Place the chicken pieces into a prepared baking dish.

4. Top the chicken with the pesto, garlic, feta cheese, and olives. Place everything into the oven to bake.

5. After 30 minutes, the dish is done and ready to eat.

## Keto Recipe #3

### *Cheese Roll-Ups*

What's in it?

- Butter (2 oz.)
- Cheddar cheese (8 oz.)

**How's it done?**

1. Take the cheese slices onto a cutting board. Slice the butter with a cheese slicer so you end up with thin slices.

2. Cover each of these slices with some butter before rolling them up and then serve and eat.

## Keto Recipe #4

### *Chicken Soup*

What's in it?

- Sliced green cabbage (2 cups)
- Shredded chicken (1.5 lbs.)

- Carrot (1)
- Chicken broth (8 cups)
- Pepper (.25 tsp.)
- Salt (1 tsp.)
- Parsley (2 tsp.)
- Minced onion (2 Tbsp.)
- Garlic cloves (2)
- Mushrooms, sliced (6 oz.)
- Celery stalks (2)
- Butter (4 oz.)

**How's it done?**

1. Start this out by melting the butter in a pot. Slice up the mushrooms and the celery into small pieces.

2. Add these to a pot along with the garlic and dried onion and cook for a few minutes.

3. After this time, add the pepper, salt, parsley, carrot, and broth. Let it all simmer until they become tender.

4. Add the cabbage and the chicken and cook for about 12 more minutes so the noodles are tender before serving.

**Keto Recipe #5**

***Keto Pizza***

What's in it?

- *Crust*
- Shredded cheese (6 oz.)
- Eggs (4)
- *Toppings*
- Salt
- Pepper
- Olive oil (4 Tbsp.)
- Leafy greens (5.5 oz.)
- Olives
- Pepperoni (1.75 oz.)
- Shredded cheese (4.25 oz.)
- Died oregano (1 tsp.)
- Tomato paste (3 Tbsp.)

**How's it done?**

1. Allow the oven to heat up to 400 degrees. While the oven warms up, take out a bowl and beat the cheese and eggs together to make the crust. Spread this out on a prepared baking sheet, making one large pizza or two small pizzas.

2. Place the pizza(s) in the oven to bake. After 15 minutes, the crust will be golden and you can take the pizza(s) out of the oven.

3. Allow the temperature of your oven to get to 450 degrees. Spread out the tomato paste on your crust and add on the rest of the toppings.

4. Place the pizza(s) back into the oven for a bit and after ten minutes, the pizza(s) should be ready. Serve with some leafy green vegetables and enjoy.

**Keto Recipe #6**

***Smoked Salmon***

What's in it?

- Pepper
- Salt
- Lime (1/2)
- Olive oil (1 Tbsp.)
- Baby spinach (2 oz.)
- Mayo (1 cup)
- Smoked salmon (.75 lbs.)

**How's it done?**

1. To start, bring out a plate and put the lime wedge, spinach, salmon and some mayo all on one plate.

2. Drizzle a bit of oil on top of the spinach before seasoning with the pepper and the salt. Serve this right away and eat.

**Keto Recipe #7**

***Mushroom Omelet***

What's in it?

- Pepper
- Salt
- Mushrooms (3)
- Yellow onion (1/3)
- Shredded cheese (1 oz.)
- Butter (1 oz.)
- Eggs (3)

**How's it done?**

1. To start this recipe, bring out a mixing bowl and crack the eggs inside. Season the eggs with pepper and salt and continue whisking to make them frothy.

2. Melt some butter in a skillet and then when it is warm, add the egg mixture.

3. When you notice this omelet is firming but is still a bit raw, add the onion, mushrooms, and cheese to the top.

4. Use a spatula to ease around the edges of your omelet so you can fold it in half. Take off the heat and serve.

**Keto Recipe #8**

***Keto Quesadillas***

What's in it?

- *Tortillas*
- Salt (1/2 tsp.)
- Coconut flour (1 Tbsp.)
- Ground psyllium husk powder (1.5 tsp.)
- Cream cheese (6 oz.)
- Egg whites (2)
- Eggs (2)
- *Filling*
- Olive oil (1 Tbsp.)
- Leafy greens (1 oz.)
- Shredded cheese (5 oz.)

**How's it done?**

1. Allow the oven to heat up to 400 degrees. While the oven is heating up, beat together your egg whites and eggs for a few minutes to make them fluffy. Add the cream cheese to your eggs and mix the cream cheese to your eggs until they are nice and smooth.

2.  In another bowl, whisk together the coconut flour, psyllium husk powder, and salt. Next, add these ingredients to your bowl of eggs and cream cheese a little at a time.

3.  When the batter is combined, let it sit for a bit so it becomes thick like pancake batter.

4.  Place two baking sheets on the counter and add parchment paper. Pour three circles of the dough on each sheet and spread into thin rounds.

5.  Next, place the two sheets of dough into the oven and let the dough cook for a bit. After five minutes, you can take the tortillas out.

6.  When the tortillas have cooled down, place them onto a cutting board and add some cheese on the tortillas. Also, add on some leafy green vegetables and the rest of the cheese on the tortilla and then top it with a second tortilla.

7.  Take out a skillet and add in some oil. Fry each of the quesadillas in the skillet for a bit on each side, letting the cheese melt.

8.  After this is done, cut up the quesadillas and then serve and eat.

**Keto Recipe #9**

*Asian Stir-Fry*

What's in it?

- Sesame oil (1 Tbsp.)

- Ginger (1 Tbsp.)

- Chili flakes (1 tsp)

- Sliced scallions (3)

- Garlic cloves (2)

- White wine vinegar (1 Tbsp.)

- Pepper (.25 tsp. or 1/4 tsp.)

- Onion powder (1 tsp.)

- Salt (1 tsp.)

- Ground beef (1.5 lbs.)

- Butter (5.5 oz.)

- Green cabbage (1.66 lbs.)

- *Wasabi Mayo*

- Wasabi paste (1 Tbsp.)

- Mayonnaise (1 cup)

**How's it done?**

1. Shred up the cabbage with your food processor. Add some butter to a frying pan and then fry your cabbage for a few minutes.

2.  Add the vinegar and spices and cook for a few more minutes before putting the cabbage in a bowl.

3.  Melt the remainder of the butter before adding the ginger, chili flakes, and garlic and then let it cook. Add the meat and let it get brown all the way through.

4.  Add the cabbage and the scallions to this mixture and stir to make it hot. Top with sesame oil, pepper, and salt.

5.  Before serving, mix the ingredients together with the mayonnaise. Serve this stir-fry with some of the wasabi mayo on top.

**Keto Recipe #10**

***Keto Pancakes***

What's in it?

- Butter (2 oz.)
- Ground psyllium husk powder (1 Tbsp.)
- Cottage cheese (7 oz.)
- Eggs (4)
- *Toppings Below*
- Whipping cream (1 cup)
- Fresh berries (8 Tbsp.)

**How's it done?**

1. To start this recipe, take out a bowl and blend all the batter ingredients together. Set the bowl to the side and let it expand for at least five minutes.

2. When you are ready, heat up a bit of the oil in a pan. Add some of the batter to the pan and let the batter cook for three minutes on both sides. Make sure to flip the batter (pancake) carefully.

3. Turn off the heat when the pancake is done and serve with the heavy cream and the berries of your choice before enjoying your meal.

# Chapter 8: The Ketogenic Diet vs. Intermittent Fasting

The ketogenic diet can be a very effective diet plan to do all on its own.

If you are able to eat the right foods and closely monitor your macronutrients, you will enter into ketosis and see big results.

Still, some people hit a rut with their weight loss goals or simply need to do even more to help improve their overall health. As a result, working with just the ketogenic diet may not be enough for some people.

One diet alternative that people can choose to practice is called intermittent fasting.

**What is Intermittent Fasting?**
Intermittent fasting is more of a lifestyle than a diet. Intermittent fasting is simply fasting or not eating food for a certain period of time.

Now that period of time of fasting or not eating food is usually between 12-16 hours. However, many people experience better results by fasting for 16 hours or more.

There are a lot of different variations when it comes to intermittent fasting, so you can choose the method that works the best for your schedule or for you to maintain for the long term.

Let's take a look at some of the basics of intermittent fasting so you can see how it will work well with the ketogenic diet.

**The Intermittent Fasting Approach**
There are actually a few different approaches that you can use when it comes to intermittent fasting.

Each intermittent fasting approach can be effective, and it is often based on what fits your schedule. The most common approaches that you can use with intermittent fasting are:

- **Skipping meals:** With this option, you will skip over a meal or two so that you can induce some extra time for fasting.

  So, for example, skipping breakfast or simply not eating in the morning can be one intermittent fasting approach.

Skipping breakfast is one of the most effective methods for practicing intermittent fasting simply because you are already fasting all night from you last meal (dinner).

If you must eat breakfast every morning than maybe try to skip either lunch and simply eat dinner.

The benefit of this intermittent fasting approach is that it allows you to experiment to see what works for you and your schedule.

- **Eating windows:** With this intermittent fasting approach, you are going to work on getting all of your macronutrients within a smaller window.

So, while most people eat from when they get up until when they go to bed, a personal practicing this intermittent fasting approach will reduce their eating time to windows of four to eight hours depending on their work and lifestyle schedules.

For example, you can have an eating window from 8:00 AM – 4:00 PM. So, this means you can only eat between 8:00 AM – 4:00 PM. So, within this eating window you can eat two or three small meals.

This intermittent fasting approach is good because you can experiment to see what is convenient for your work and lifestyle schedules.

- **One to two-day cleanses:** With this intermittent fasting approach, you are going to put yourself on an extended fasting period.

  With one to two-day cleanses, you will simply avoid eating for one or two days. You can do one or two-day cleanses once or twice a week.

  Now this intermittent fasting approach will effectively reduce the number of calories that you consume resulting in great weight loss.

Most people will find that it is hard to start out with a one or two day fast, which is why restricting your eating window or skipping meals are two of the best intermittent fasting approaches you can choose from.

Remember to experiment with intermittent fasting and try out different eating windows for a week or so to see what intermittent fasting approach works best for you.

## How Does Intermittent Fasting Work?

While there are a few different options when it comes to choosing an intermittent fasting approach, you may wonder why it can be so effective.

The whole point of intermittent fasting is to simply eat food during a certain period of time.

Our bodies will only be able to take in so much food at once, so if we are only allowed to eat for a few hours during the day and then fast during the rest, we are limiting our calorie intake which results in weight loss.

During the fasting time, we are not allowed to eat at all.

Our metabolism also seems to speed up as long as the fasting period is short, such as fasting for just eighteen hours rather than for a whole week or more.

So not only are we reducing the calories that we are able to consume because our bodies can't take in that much food at one time, we are also speeding up our metabolism at the same time.

Over time, your body is going to learn how to adjust to intermittent fasting.

In the beginning, intermittent fasting is going to be hard and you may feel hungry during the fasting period. But if you can maintain your periods of fasting, the body will eventually adapt and you will be able to feel just fine without eating all day long.

In addition, maintaining your periods of fasting and keeping track of the food you eat will eventually become easier when you only have a few hours a day to eat.

It is important to state that when you are in a fasting state, the body is able to break down some of the extra fat that is being stored by your body.

Now if you include ketosis from the ketogenic diet, all of the excess fat that you have on your body will simply melt off in no time. In addition, you will still have plenty of energy for all of your daily activities.

Ketosis actually mimics the fasting state because we take the glucose out of our bloodstream so that we can use fats as our main source of energy.

During your fast, the body is going to rely on those extra fat stores to help you to stay energized.

If you are doing intermittent fasting along with the ketogenic diet, you need to make sure that you really get the sufficient amount of fat content that the body needs so that the body can get the right amounts of energy that it needs.

It is important to state that when you combine both intermittent fasting and the ketogenic diet together, you will be able to burn through fat, lower your glucose levels, and see tremendous results in your overall health.

Intermittent fasting is not necessarily for weight loss, although it can help you to lose weight if you are prone to overeating throughout the day.

In addition, intermittent fasting can help you reduce your calorie intake resulting in weight loss.

When you combine intermittent fasting with the ketogenic diet, you are sure to see some tremendous weight loss results as well as an increase in your health benefits.

**Are the Ketogenic Diet and Intermittent Fasting Similar?**
There are a few similarities that you will find with the ketogenic diet and intermittent fasting.

Both are going to work to limit the amount of glucose in your diet so that the body will start to rely more on using fats for energy rather than carbs and sugars for energy. This is an effective way to melt the fat off your body and help you to lose weight.

However, the methods that both use to help you reach this result are different.

The ketogenic diet helps you to use fat as energy by changing up the macronutrients that you consume to cut out the carbs. Intermittent fasting will help you to burn fat because you will be forced to reduce how many calories you are able to consume as a result of having a small eating window.

The ketogenic diet is an eating plan. With the ketogenic diet you have certain foods that you are able to consume, and you need to stick with eating those specific foods if you want to be on this diet plan.

On the other hand, intermittent fasting can be done with any type of diet plan. However, intermittent fasting will not be effective if you only eat junk food during your eating window.

But you can combine intermittent fasting with other diets such as the Mediterranean diet, or any other diet plan that you choose.

But when intermittent fasting is combined with the ketogenic diet, you are going to get some amazing weight loss results and your overall health will greatly improve.

**Can I Use Intermittent Fasting and the Ketogenic Diet Together?**
Yes, it is possible to use both intermittent fasting and the ketogenic diet together.

Keep in mind, intermittent fasting is more about fasting or not eating for a certain period of time each and every day and that period of time can be between 12-16 hours or more.

Now the ketogenic diet is more about the types of foods that you would eat each and every day specifically low carbs, a lot of healthy fats and moderate protein.

It is important to state that you do not have to go on an intermittent fasting diet in order to lose weight with the ketogenic diet.

It is already hard enough for many people to follow the ketogenic diet so combining both intermittent fasting and the ketogenic diet for weight loss is not required, but instead an option.

But for those people who would like to experiment and seek to achieve their weight loss goals and improve their overall health, then combining both intermittent fasting and the ketogenic diet is definitely a great idea.

With intermittent fasting, you will limit the hours that you are able to eat. Instead of allowing yourself to spread your meals and your snacks all throughout the day, you will limit your "eating window" to just a few hours a day.

With intermittent fasting, many people will choose to only eat between 10:00 AM - 6:00 PM and eat all of their macronutrients during this time period. Others will do a whole day of fasting once or twice a week where they are not allowed to eat at all for one full day.

When people do a full day of fasting they try to consume all of their nutrients on the other days of the week in order to have sufficient energy for their one full day of fasting.

Just keep in mind that the point of intermittent fasting is that you are limiting the amount of time that you are able to eat which forces you to eat fewer calories which results in weight loss.

Now if you ever feel like you hit a plateau with your weight loss goals while on the ketogenic diet, simply consider combining the ketogenic diet with intermittent fasting.

Combining both the ketogenic diet and intermittent fasting will definitely "shock" the body and you will also benefit greatly by burning more fat and achieving your weight loss goals.

When you combine intermittent fasting with the ketogenic diet, you must remember to stick with the macronutrients that we discussed above that are approved for the ketogenic diet.

So, you will still stick with a high fat, moderate protein, and low carb diet plan even while intermittent fasting.

You will just need to be more careful about the times you eat those macronutrients, but otherwise, you can follow the ketogenic diet exactly the same.

If you want to get some of the benefits that come with intermittent fasting or you want to increase your weight loss, then combining intermittent fasting with the ketogenic diet can be very effective.

You can experiment with the different types of intermittent fasting variations that are available to see which one fits into your schedule and works best for you.

Of course, if you find the ketogenic diet is effective enough or adding in intermittent fasting is too difficult, you can always just stay with the ketogenic diet on its own and still see some amazing results.

# Conclusion

Thank you for making it through the end of this book. I hope the book was educational, informative and able to provide you with all of the tools you need to achieve your health and weight loss goals or whatever they may be.

The next step is to get started with the ketogenic diet. This is one of the most effective diet plans that is available for helping you to lose weight.

While you will need to get used to some of the dietary changes that are unusual compared to other traditional diet plans, the ketogenic diet will really help you to lose weight in no time.

So, what you have come to learn from this book is what exactly the ketogenic diet is all about and how you can use it for your own weight loss journey.

You have learned the basics of the ketogenic diet, the benefits of trying it out, how you can use it with intermittent fasting to lose more weight, the foods that are allowed on the ketogenic diet, and even some meal plans to help you get started.

It is important to mention that the more information that you have before starting the ketogenic diet, the more you will be successful with this diet.

Just keep in mind that when you are tired of trying out all the other diet plans that haven't been successful in the past and you want to work with something that will actually work, the ketogenic diet is always a great option for weight loss.

Finally, if you found this book useful in any way, a review on Amazon is always appreciated!

Thanks, and I wish you great success with the ketogenic diet.

# SPECIAL BONUS!

One last thing before you go.  You have access to free additional information regarding living a Health and Fitness Lifestyle.

The following Health and Fitness information is very different than the usual "Get a Six Pack," or "Build Strong Muscles."

Instead, the following information will simply improve your overall wellbeing.

Please continue reading on the following page and enjoy.

# Additional Chapters

## Sleep Benefits for Weight Loss

Every busy person has a shortage of time. However, when it comes to sleep, you must make time for getting enough sleep in order to succeed in business and in life.

There are so many benefits to exercise and having a healthy diet. But when it truly comes to weight loss, sleep is the secret to fat loss and here is why…

### Sleep Controls Your Diet and Fitness Lifestyle

Believe it or not but sleep is more important than diet and exercise.

The reason why sleep is more important than diet and exercise is because if you don't get enough sleep (7-9 hours) every night, your lack of sleep will negatively affect both your diet and your fitness goals.

Research shows that the more you sleep the more weight you lose because you will have the energy and focus to stick to your diet as well as to exercise with tremendous energy.

This concept of sleeping more to lose more weight is very simple yet very difficult to follow by many people especially busy entrepreneurs. The solution is to make sleep a priority just like accomplishing your entrepreneurial goals are a priority.

**Sleep Eliminates Food Cravings**

Research shows that getting enough sleep eliminates food cravings because your body is not stressed from a lack of a good night's sleep. However, when you don't get enough sleep, you cause your body to develop stress.

When you are stressed, this hormone called cortisol causes you to crave food especially unhealthy foods and what happens is that eventually you give in and begin to eat more and more.

Cortisol is responsible for weight gain so whenever your body produces cortisol, you will simply gain weight.

In order to prevent cortisol from developing in the body, you have to make sure you are getting enough sleep.

It does not matter how much you exercise or how strict your diet is. If you do not get enough sleep, your body will be craving food as a result of the stress it undergoes as a result of not getting enough sleep.

## Good Sleep Builds Muscle

If you strength train and get a good night's sleep you allow your body to repair itself. In addition, you allow your body to build muscle as a result of getting a good night's sleep.

Building muscle is good for fighting fat because even if you have small amounts of muscle, this muscle will force your body to burn off calories.

## Sleep is the Fountain of Youth

Whenever you get a good night's rest, your body develops Human Growth Hormone (HGH).

Human growth Hormone is a natural hormone that your body develops and is responsible for anti-aging.

More specifically, Human Growth Hormone enhances weight loss, develops stronger bones, builds muscle, reduces cardiovascular disease, improves your mood and improves your cognitive function.

Therefore, the more you sleep, the more Human Growth Hormone your body will develop. As a result, you will live longer and feel more youthful and energetic as a result of sleeping more.

**Sleep Gives You Superior Energy**

When you get a good night of sleep, you wake up feeling refreshed ready to take on the world. In addition, you will be more motivated to exercise, eat healthy and accomplish your daily goals as a result of getting a good night's sleep.

It is also important to state that getting a good night's sleep will give you razor sharp focus and a strong willingness to accomplish your daily goals especially your entrepreneurial goals.

**The More You Sleep the Less You Eat**

Research shows that the earlier you go to sleep and the more you sleep (7-9 hours), the less likely you are to eat because you will be eliminating late night snacking and boredom from staying up late.

In addition, sleeping more will help to keep you focus on your diet and exercise routine as a result of being well rested.

**Sleeping More Burns More Calories**

Research shows that you burn more calories when you sleep between 7-9 hours per night then if you were to sleep between 4-6 hours per night.

The reason being is because when you sleep 7-9 hour per night, your body is working more efficiently at burning calories as a result of it being well rested.

However, if you only sleep between 4-6 hours per night, your body will be under tremendous stress and will feel lethargic making your body to burn less calories over time.

**A Good Night Sleep Will Help You to Shop for Healthy Foods**
Research shows that people that get a good night's rest are likelier to eat healthier as well as shop for healthier food versus people that don't get enough sleep.

This is because people that don't get enough sleep tend to drink sugary drinks like coffee with extra sugar and energy drinks in order to stay awake.

In addition, a person that does not get a good night's rest will be stressed out and will be searching for comfort foods which most likely will be unhealthy foods.

**Here are Some Tips for a Better Night's Sleep**
- Turn off your computer, cell phone, and TV at least 30 minutes before you go to sleep.

- Make your bed and bedroom as relaxing as possible in order to ensure a good night's sleep.

- Create a nightly bedtime ritual. Consider taking a warm bath or reading a book before going to bed. In addition, eliminate doing any important work before going to bed.

- Develop a bedtime schedule. Figure out what time you want to wake up in the morning then decide to go to sleep every night at the same time making sure you sleep between 7-9 hours every night.

- Eliminate drinking any fluids before you go to sleep in order to prevent waking up at night to go to the toilet. In addition, eliminate drinking coffee early in the evening and stay away from energy drinks, soda and alcohol if possible.

- Try to sleep in complete darkness if possible. If this is uncomfortable consider buying a lamp with a timer that shuts off after a few minutes.

# What is the Best Home Exercise Equipment for Busy People?

The answer is simple…there is no best home exercise equipment. However, there is a lot great home exercise equipment that many people can benefit from.

But think of health and fitness like this…if you are a busy person that likes to exercise from home, then there are a lot of variety of training equipment that you can use to workout at home.

**Here are some good examples of exercise equipment for training at home:**

**Chair Gym**

A chair gym is a convenient light weight resistance chair that allows you to do total body workouts while sitting on a chair. The chair gym allows you to work out your abs, legs, arms and shoulders all from a seated position.

The chair gym is a great piece of training equipment for strengthening the entire body. In addition, the chair gym is very safe because you can do a lot of low impact but effective exercises.

**Standing Desk**

A standing desk is great if you want to do some very light exercise at home while you stand up and do some work on your computer.

A standing desk will help you eliminate lower back pain as well as stiffness and soreness you may feel from sitting down on a chair at a traditional desk for long periods of time.

A standing desk is great because it allows you to stretch out your legs and lower body while you work on your computer.

**Desk Treadmill**

Desk Treadmills are great because they allow you to walk while you work on your laptop computer.

Desk treadmill are so convenient because they are inexpensive, small and there are all kinds of styles.

In addition, desk treadmills don't take a lot of space because there are desk treadmills that even fit under your desk.

Desk treadmills make for a great exercise tool for training at home because you can transition from walking to running.

Overall, desk treadmills are very convenient for getting a great workout at home.

## Wobble Chairs

Wobble chairs are great because they provide motion for your lower back. Wobble chairs work by allowing your lower back to safely move in different positions. In addition, wobble chairs provide flexibility to the lower back and reduce lower back pain as a result of their ability to safely move around.

Wobble chairs are also great because they provide proper circulation throughout the body and they safely allow for stretching of tight and sore lower body muscles.

## Desk Cycle Pedal Exerciser

A desk cycle pedal exerciser is great for home entrepreneur's because it allows you to workout your legs while sitting down and doing work at a desk.

Desk pedal exercisers are also great because they help to keep the blood flowing in the body. In addition, they workout the largest muscles of the body which are the legs. They also help you to do some cardiovascular exercise which is great for the heart.
Desk pedal exercisers are also great for reducing lower body stiffness and soreness. Desk pedal exercisers are also great because they help to burn additional calories.

Desk pedal exercisers are also easy to use because they can be placed under a desk and they don't take up a lot of space.

## FitDesk Bike

A FitDesk Bike also known as a Workstation Exercise Bike is similar to a stationary bike but it has a work station where you can comfortably put your laptop computer on it so that you can do some work while you pedal away.

A FitDesk Bike is a great way to get some exercise all while conveniently reading, writing or simply doing some work on a computer.

Another benefit of a FitDesk Bike is that the seats are very comfortable and the overall design of the bike provides more flexibility and movement than sitting on a traditional chair.

FitDesk Bikes are inexpensive and there are different kinds of FitDesk Bikes that you can choose from so check them out!

## Desk Monitor and Laptop Mounts

Desk monitor mounts are great because they can be mounted to a traditional desk or wall and can be used as a standing desk.

There are also desk laptop mounts that can be used for placing a laptop on in order to do some work.

Both desk monitor and laptop mounts are convenient because they do not take up space and they can be used at work or at home.

Both desk monitor and laptop mounts are great for allowing a person to alternate between sitting down and standing up. In addition, desk monitor and laptop mounts help a person to reduce lower back pain as well as soreness and cramps from sitting down at a traditional desk.

**Wobble Boards**

Wobble boards also known as standing desk balance boards or rockers are used when standing up at a standing desk.

All you do is simply stand on this small board at your standing desk and you balance yourself. Before you know it, you will be moving back and forth in a rocking motion.

What is great about wobble boards is that if you want to change from simply standing up straight at a standing desk you can simply stand on a wobble board at your standing desk.

**Some of the benefits of using a wobble board are:**
- You will move more than simply standing at a standing desk.
- You can work comfortable on your computer while standing on a wobble board.
- You will be getting some exercise while you are balancing yourself back and forth on your wobble board.

- You will be getting more movement throughout your lower body as a result of using a wobble board.
- You will be very alert as a result of balancing back and forth on a wobble board.
- Wobble boards are fun to stand on!

## Kneeling Chairs

Kneeling chairs have nothing to do with kneeling on the floor. Instead, kneeling chairs are awesome because they are specialized chairs that force you to sit upright.

In addition, when you sit on a kneeling chair, you don't have to think about sitting upright because the chair is specially designed for you to naturally keep your spin in a neutral position which keeps you sitting upright.

Kneeling chairs are great because they reduce lower back pain. In addition, kneeling chairs improve your posture because they are designed to have you sit upright which forces you to have good posture.

## Fitbit Trackers

Fitbit Trackers are these sporty athletic watches that are great because they show you how many steps you take in a day. In addition, FitBit Trackers allow you to compete against other people in FitBit groups to see who has walked the most in a day.

FitBit Trackers can also motivate you to move more on a daily basis because they teach you to be accountable for your health and fitness lifestyle.

In addition, FitBit Trackers allow you to monitor your heart rate as well as track your sleep which is also great for improving your health.  A FitBit Tracker will even help you to feel better because you will be motivated to move more every day.

# How to Get Fit and Stay Fit from Home

Whether you are a busy entrepreneur working from home or an office worker, here are some great tips to help you get fit and stay fit from home:

### Remove All Junk Food from Your Home

Simply, remove all junk food from your home and instead replace these unhealthy foods with healthy snacks. Some healthy snacks to eat are fruits and healthy nuts like almonds, walnuts and cashes and you can even eat some dark chocolate!

If you are a busy entrepreneur that works from an office, consider taking healthy snacks to your office instead of buying unhealthy foods and snacks on the way to work.

### Use a Comfortable Chair to Sit On

As a busy entrepreneur you may be required to sit down for long hours. However, it is important to use a comfortable chair to sit on in order to eliminate any discomfort you may face from sitting on a hard, uncomfortable chair.

At the moment there are all kinds of comfortable chairs that you can use for your home or work office. In addition, these comfortable chairs will definitely help eliminate any pain or discomfort you may face from using an uncomfortable chair.

## Use A Standing Desk

Say you get a comfortable chair and your body still feels a little tired and sore from sitting down for long hours. What you can do instead is to use a standing desk.

A Standing desk is a great way to stand and stretch out your legs, back and overall lower body while you continue to do important work at the same time.

## Alternate Sitting and Standing Throughout the Day

You can even alternate between sitting on a comfortable chair for 30 minutes and then switching to a standing desk for another 30 minutes. Then you can give your entire body and mind a 10-minute break from all of your hard work.

## Take A Break Every Hour

Simply take a break every hour and get your body moving. You can take a break for 10-15 minutes and maybe do some light stretching or you can even do some dynamic stretches like arm and leg circles as well as hip and waist rotations.

You can even do some easy bodyweight exercises like pushups, bodyweight squats or lunges to get the blood flowing in your body.

**Use A Foam Roller**

Foam rollers are great for giving yourself a personal massage. In addition, foam rollers can be used to relieve any soreness or tightness you may feel throughout your body.

Foam rollers are also great for improving flexibility and mobility. So instead of spending money on getting an expensive massage, simply invest in a foam roller and reek all the benefits a foam roller has to offer.

**Set A Schedule and Develop Discipline to Stick to It**

Some people are morning people and others are night owls. Do whatever works best for you. However, develop the habit of creating a work, eating and fitness schedule and stick to it so that you can make sure you are living a healthy lifestyle while pursuing your entrepreneurial goals.

In addition, developing a work, eating and fitness schedule will keep you focused on what is important and what you should focus on as well as what your priorities are.

You will also be more organized if you develop a work, eating and fitness schedule and stick to it than if you had no plan whatsoever.

**Create a Fitness Social Club**

Whether you are a solo entrepreneur or you work from your busy work office, set out to create a small fitness social club where you can meet other like-minded individuals and workout together.

You can even include your colleagues as a part of a "fitness meeting" where you can share ideas and discuss work issues all while working out together.

**Create a Healthy Environment**

Whether you work from home or from your work office, create an environment that is relaxing and enjoyable for you.

You can look into getting some home/office fitness gear such as a work desk to make sure you are moving your body or you can even use a gym chair which provides a total body workout.

You can also consider getting a tower fan which will keep you cool whether at your home or work office. If you work from home, you can even consider getting a cycling work station or a under desk treadmill for the purpose of getting some exercise while you work at the same time.

**Practicing Intermittent Fasting**

Intermittent Fasting is a great way to safely lose weight and keep it off permanently. In addition, intermittent fasting will give you a clear mind to focus on your busy work projects all while losing fat.

Intermittent fasting will prevent you from constantly eating so much as a result of following an eating schedule.

Intermittent fasting will give you the freedom to work more and do more and focus less on eating as a result of reducing the number of meals you eat per day.

Intermittent fasting has so many benefits that EVERY busy entrepreneur should make it part of their busy lives.

**Drink Lots of Water**

Forget all the coffee, juice and soda and stick to drinking lots and lots of water.

Water will keep you feeling full and prevent you from feeling fatigue from dehydration. In addition, drinking water especially cold water will increase your metabolism which will make you burn more calories. Water is also good for the skin and will give you more energy to do more as well.

## Sleep More

According to research, sleep is more important than nutrition and exercise.

Lack of sleep will reduce your mental and physical performance. In addition, lack of sleep will develop stress in your body causing you to gain weight. Lack of sleep will also affect your mood and hormones.

As you can see, you want to make sure you sleep as much as possible especially if you are a busy entrepreneur working long hours day after day, week after week.

Sleep is extremely beneficial for being a successful entrepreneur because it will repair your body and mind from all the mental and physical stress you put it through day after day so make sure you are getting lots and lots of sleep.

## Plan Your Meals and Eat the Same Meals

Plan your meals ahead. You can also develop the habit of eating the same healthy foods every day both for lunch and dinner. This keeps shopping for healthy foods easy and it is an efficient way of eating because you will develop the habit of shopping for and cooking the same foods every day.

## Use a Food Scale

Use a food scale to weigh your food before you cook it so that you know exactly how much food you will be consuming every day both for lunch and dinner.

By using a food scale, you will be able to keep track of the number of calories you are eating every day. In addition, you will be more efficient at losing weight because you will not be overeating as a result of keeping track of how much food you eat.

Research shows that 80% of weight loss is all about your diet and what you eat and how much you eat.

So, by weighing your food, you will know if you need to reduce the number of calories you are eating in order to lose weight. In addition, weighing your food will help you to maintain your desired weight.

# How to Exercise and Stay in Shape While Traveling

If you are traveling for business or pleasure and you want to exercise and stay in shape, what do you do?

When do you workout?

Where do you workout?

How do you workout?

What equipment do you use?

What kind of workouts do you do?

What foods do you eat?

Sometimes it is hard to workout and stay in shape while traveling because our normal exercise routines and eating habits get thrown out the window when traveling. However, it is very possible to workout, eat healthy and stay in shape while traveling.

If you travel but feel that you don't know how to workout and stay in shape while traveling, then you have nothing to worry about.

Here are some great tips, action plans and even exercise routines that you can use as a guide while traveling:

## Use A Hotel's Resources

When staying at a resort or hotel, ask the front desk if there is an available exercise gym or training facility for its customers.

In addition, you can even ask the resort/hotel if it has a swimming pool where you can go for a swim.

Many hotels offer weight machines, treadmills, stationary bicycles, and fitness mats for stretching or exercising.

Ask hotel staff where the fitness center is located in the building and what the hours are for the facility.

Sometimes, hotels and resorts may even have an office that organizes bicycle tours, hiking trips, walking tours and other fitness adventures so make sure to ask your resort/hotel for more details.

## Stay Active at The Airport

Most of the time you will arrive early to the Airport.  Usually, you will arrive between 1-3 hours before your flight departs.

Well, you don't have to just check-in with the airlines and sit down for 1-2 hours and wait for your flight to depart.

Instead, you can stand up, walk around the airport and get some exercise while you wait for your flight to depart.

You can simply walk around the airport and do some "people watching." You can also walk around the airport and do some window shopping stopping by all the small shops that are located within the airport.

To get a better workout, you can walk with your small carry-on backpack throughout the airport.

The extra resistance that the carry-on backpack has to offer will strengthen your legs, core, shoulders and overall body as a result of carrying extra weight.

Once it is time to board your flight, you can now sit-down and get some rest.

**Avoid Airport Food**

Whatever you do, don't eat at the airport!

First, the food at the airport is very expensive!

Next, most of the time the food at the airport is very unhealthy.

If you must eat food at the airport then simply plan ahead and bring some healthy snacks with you.

For example, you can bring some easy to carry fruit with you like a banana, an apple or an orange.

You can also bring some healthy unsalted nuts with you like walnuts, almonds or cashews.

**Avoid Airplane Food**
I know, I know you have to eat.
But one thing about airplane food is that it is not very healthy.
But consider this…what about bringing your own healthy food on the plane?

In addition to bringing some healthy snacks with you on the plane, you can also bring with you some tuna lunch kits.

Tuna lunch kits are small packets of dried tuna (usually in a small can) that are packaged with unsalted crackers.

Tuna lunch kits are great because they are small to carry, they are allowed to be brought onto the airplane and they are healthy for you!

Depending on how far you are traveling, you can bring two or three of these healthy tuna lunch kits with you.

If you really want to challenge yourself you can simply skip eating all together while flying and simply practice intermittent fasting until you arrive to your destination!

## Use a Fitness App

Research show that people that use fitness apps are likelier to remain consistent with their health and fitness lifestyle then people that don't use fitness apps.

In addition, research also shows that people that use fitness apps are more active then people that don't use fitness apps.

As you can see, fitness apps are great for keeping you in shape while you travel.

In addition, there are all kinds of fitness apps that you can use from running apps to strength training apps to yoga apps to even nutrition apps.

As you can see, fitness apps are great for making sure you stay consistent with your health and fitness lifestyle.

## Use a FitBit Tracker

A FitBit Tracker is a fitness gadget that monitors your eating habits, your fitness workouts and keeps track of how many hours of sleep you get every night.

In addition, a FitBit Tracker will keep you motivated to exercise more by showing you EXACTLY how many miles you have walked in a day as well as how many calories you have burned and even how much water you drank.

Using a FitBit Tracker is a great way to stay motived to exercise more and stay consistent with your health and fitness goals while you travel.

**Swim at The Hotel's Pool**
If the hotel or resort you are staying at has a swimming pool, then take advantage of this luxury.

Swimming is an excellent form of exercise. You can get a great workout by swimming laps back and forth.

But what if you don't know how to swim?

No problem. You can simply walk back and forth in the shallow end of the pool for 20-30 minutes and you can still get a great workout.

In addition, you can even do some low impact running in the shallow end of the pool.

You can also do some strength training exercises in the shallow end of the pool like jumping squats, jumping jacks, knee raises and more!

The variety of exercises that you can do in a swimming pool are endless. So, pack your swimsuit and ask your hotel to see if they have a pool and if they do, jump right in!!!

**Walk Around Your Hotel**

You can get a great workout by simply walking around the hotel or even within the hotel you are staying at.

You can look for a flight of stairs where you can walk up and down or maybe even run a couple of flights of stairs for strength, endurance and power.

You can even go for a jog around your hotel but it all depends on you to use your creative mind to get a good workout at the hotel or resort you are staying at.

In addition, personal motivation plays a key role in make sure you exercise, eat healthy and get in shape while traveling.

**Follow The 80/20 Rule**

The 80/20 Rule is fun and simple and can be applied to anything in life.

The 80/20 Rule works like this: **80% of the time eat healthy and 20% of the time eat unhealthily or anything you want.** That's it!

For example, you have a healthy lunch that consists of oatmeal with a banana and some egg whites.  You then decide to have a small piece of chocolate for dessert.

So, 80% of your lunch was healthy because it consisted of nutritious oatmeal with a banana and egg whites. But 20% of your lunch was unhealthy because you ate a small piece of chocolate for dessert.

Nevertheless, as long as 80% of the time you are eating healthy, then that is all that matters when it comes to the 80/20 Rule.

If you follow the 80/20 Rule, you will most likely succeed at staying fit and healthy while traveling.

You have to remember that we are all human and that we all crave delicious foods especially when we travel.

So, the next time you travel, keep the 80/20 Rule in mind for making sure you remain consistent with your health and fitness goals.

**Rent A Bicycle**

There are many cities around the world that allow tourists to rent a bicycle.

In addition, renting a bicycle can be an economical way of exploring a new destination while getting some exercise.

You can also combine riding a bicycle with walking which makes for an excellent workout!

And when you get tired of riding your bicycle, you can simply sit down somewhere that is scenic and get some rest while you enjoy the beautiful view.

I remember when I first went to Europe I rented a bicycle in Barcelona, Spain. Wow, that experience was great!

Don't be afraid of renting a bicycle when you travel to another city.

Many cities around the world have friendly bicycle lanes for tourists and riders to ride their bicycles on.

So, get out there, rent a bicycle for an hour or two, explore a new destination and get some exercise!

**Practice Intermittent Fasting**
Intermittent fasting is a great way to stay in shape while traveling.

If you are not sure what to eat while traveling simply stick to eating two meals (specifically lunch and dinner) a day while fasting in order to make sure you do not eat too many calories.

In addition, you can even indulge in some of the local cuisine while practicing intermittent fasting and still stay in shape.

**Run Outside**

Running is a great way to exercise and stay in shape while traveling.

All you have to do is pack your running shoes and run outside. That's it!

You can look for the nearest park or trails to run at. But simply just get out there and run and enjoy the beautiful scenery.

**Free Outdoor Gyms**

Some cities around the world have outdoor training gyms that are FREE and all you have to do is simply show up and exercise.

Some training gyms are at a beach and some are located at parks but the outdoor training gyms are available for everyone to use.

Usually the outdoor gyms will consist of a lot of pull-up bars, parallel dip bars, monkey bars and other bodyweight equipment for you to use.

However, some outdoor gyms come equipped with elliptical machines, exercise bikes and various other kinds of exercise machines.

So, the next time you plan to travel, consider working out at a FREE outdoor gym.

**Change Up Your Workout Routine**

When you travel to a new destination, don't be afraid to try new exercises as well as new exercise equipment.

I remember when I first went to live in South Korea for work, the city I was living in didn't seem to have any fitness gyms near my home.

But what I did find was that there were a bunch of trails to go off-road running. In addition, I also found a bunch of outdoor calisthenics playgrounds where I would go and do a bunch of bodyweight exercises.

I have to say I truly miss running on the trails in South Korea as well as working out at the outdoor calisthenics playgrounds.

So, keep this in mind…if you travel to a new destination and there is a lack of equipment that you are used to using, simply adapt to the environment and use what is available.

Don't be afraid to try new exercise equipment or to do new exercises when you travel.

In addition, you can experiment with developing new exercise routines and programs as well as with eating new kinds of healthy foods.

Remember, adapt to the environment, stay focused on your fitness goals and get fit!

**Get in Shape in Your Hotel Room**

If there is no gym at your hotel or near your hotel, then take it upon yourself to exercise in your hotel room.

I remember when I moved from the U.S. to China 3 years ago, I didn't know where to find a gym to exercise. So, what I did was I simply exercised in my hotel room.

I started by warming up doing some easy body weight exercises like pushups, bodyweight squats and lunges.

I then moved on doing more challenging exercises like pushup burpees and handstand pushups using the wall.

Let me tell you I was still able to get a great workout inside my hotel room.

Keep in mind that you can do a variety of challenging bodyweight workouts in your hotel room.  In addition, no equipment is needed for getting a good workout from your hotel room. The only thing that is need is your creativity in order to get an effective workout.

**Here is a simple workout routine that you can do inside your hotel room:**

<u>**Bodyweight Circuit Routine (4-6 sets)**</u>
- Bodyweight Squats (12-15 repetitions)
- Pushups (10 -12 repetitions)
- Sit-ups (12-15 repetitions)
- Mountain climbers (10-12 repetitions)
- Jumping Jacks (30 repetitions)

**Run in place for 30 seconds*

***Rest 30 seconds and repeat circuit*

Remember, there are so many exercises you can do from within your hotel room. You can do burpees or jump rope all from your hotel room. Just remember that all of these exercises will give you a great workout when there is no gym around.

**Do Some Yoga or Stretching**

Doing yoga or some stretching while traveling are great ways to stay in shape.

You can easily do some yoga or stretching in your very own hotel room but if there is an exercise gym within your hotel that is even better.

Yoga and simply stretching are good for developing flexibility throughout the body. In addition, Yoga and stretching help to develop a better posture.

Yoga and stretching are also great stress relievers and help to alleviate back pain and soreness from sitting down for long periods of time.

Simply yoga and stretching will help to relieve the tension from traveling while working your muscles and toning your core.

**Pack Lightweight Exercise Equipment**

If you are able to plan your workouts in advance before you travel, you can try packing some exercise equipment that will fit in your luggage without adding excessive weight or bulk.

For example, you can bring a light jump rope or some resistance bands with you on your travels.

You can also consider bringing a small foam roller to help alleviate any soreness from traveling.

You can also consider bringing your swimsuit and goggles in case there is a swimming pool for you to swim.

## Go Golfing

Golfing may not sound like a very intense workout to some people.

However, golf does require a lot of walking. In addition, you get to enjoy the outdoors in a very peaceful environment away from all the stress of a busy city. In addition, golfing can be a great way to relax.

There are so many great places around the world that have beautiful golf courses. So, if you are traveling to a new destination and you like golf, look into taking the time to play a few games of golf.

## Frisbee, Tennis or Play Catch

If you are traveling with family or friends, consider taking with you a small frisbee or a small ball to throw around with one another.

You can maybe even brink some tennis rackets for playing tennis. You can even pack a baseball glove and a ball so that you play catch outside.

Like I said before, be creative and use your creative mind for getting fit while traveling.

**Explore the City by Foot**

Before you travel, do some research on the internet regarding your destination. Look for some places that would be of interest to you and go explore those places by foot.

You can simply walk throughout the city seeing new sites and meeting new people all by foot. If you get tired, simply jump in a taxi or take the train back to your hotel.

Walking is a great form of exercise and you can do it anywhere and anytime. Just make sure to bring with you a good pair of walking shoes.

**Go Dancing**

Have you ever looked at a professional dancer's body?

Dancers have amazing bodies because of all the movement they are doing with their bodies.

I know that some cities during the summer have FREE outdoor dance classes where tourists and locals can participate.

I personally know that my hometown, Chicago, has many free outdoor dance classes available to the public during the summer season.

You can participate in a variety of dance classes from salsa dancing to tango to swing dancing to even hip-hop dancing.
``

If you want to go dancing at your new destination, all you have to do is ask the reception desk at your hotel if they know of any places where you can go dancing.

You can also ask the reception desk for an events brochure of the city you are visiting to see if there are any places where you can go dancing. So, don't be shy, get on the dance floor!

**Eat Healthy Foods**
Staying in shape while traveling may sometimes not be the easiest thing to do.

There are so many varieties of delicious foods to eat especially when you travel to foreign countries.

However, if you stick to the basics like eating fruits, vegetables and lean meats, you will have better success with staying in shape while traveling.

In addition, don't be afraid to shop at a local supermarket for healthy snacks and fruits.

You can even try some of the local fruit like the exotic Durian fruit in Thailand and the Dragon Fruit in China.

**Make a Commitment to Exercise**

It is important to be consistent with getting some exercise while you travel.  Simply, don't make excuses for not be able to exercise while traveling.

Instead do whatever it takes to get some exercise every day and that can be from running outside to doing some bodyweight exercises in your hotel room.

No matter what, have a fitness plan before you travel and be consistent with your training schedule.

**Do Full Body Workouts**

To make sure you are exercising your entire body while traveling, try to focus on doing full body workouts.

Full body workouts are great because you will exercise the entire body in a short amount of time. In addition, the exercises can be done in your hotel room, at a gym or even outside!

**Here are some circuit routines for a Full Body Workout:**
<u>**Circuit Routine 1 (4-6 Sets)**</u>
- Bodyweight squats (12-15) repetitions

- Pushups (8-12) repetitions
- Sit-ups (10-15) repetitions
  *rest 1minute

## Circuit Routine 2 (4-6 Sets)

- Lunges (alternate forward and reverse) (12-15) repetitions
- Diamond Pushups (8-12) repetitions
- Bodyweight planks (30-45 seconds)
  *rest 1minute

## Circuit Routine 3 (4-6 Sets)

- Pushup Burpees (6-8) repetitions
- Flutter kicks (12-15 repetitions)
- Mountain climbers (10-12 repetitions)
- *rest 1minute

**Keep Track of Your Fitness Goals**

Keep a journal of your fitness goals whenever you travel. You can do so by writing down your workouts and your progress.

In addition, keep a food journal. Try to write down what you ate and what time you ate especially if you are practicing intermittent fasting.

**Prioritize Your Diet**

Although exercise is great for the body, mind and spirit, when it comes to losing weight, it is all about your DIET.

Simply to be lean and stay in shape you really have to focus on your diet.  So, if you can really focus on your diet in addition to getting some daily exercise while you travel, you will be able to remain fit 365 days a year.

To make sure you are staying in shape while traveling, make every attempt to eat a lot of fruits, vegetables, nuts and lean meats.

You can also consider shopping at the local supermarket to make sure that the food you are buying is fresh.

If you include practicing intermittent fasting while traveling along with doing some daily exercise, you will be sure to retain your athletic figure no matter where you travel around the world.

So, combine intermittent fasting, with eating some healthy food and getting some daily exercise while traveling and you will be able to get fit and stay fit along your travel journeys.

**Develop Some Fitness Goals**
Before you travel, develop some fitness goals you want to achieve while traveling.

For example, if you are traveling to a city that has a lot of mountains, then consider making hiking one of your fitness goals.

If you are traveling to a big city like Hong Kong or London, then consider exploring the city by foot or by bicycle if possible.

If you are traveling to a city that has beautiful beaches and you always wanted to take surfing lessons, then plan for this!

So, before you leave home create some fitness goals you want to accomplish while you travel. This way you will be likelier to stick to your health and fitness lifestyle.

**Don't Forget to Drink Water!**
It is easy to forget to drink eight glasses (or more) of water per day whenever you travel.

But if you want to stay hydrated, fit and healthy you have to remember to drink lots of water daily.

Simply by drinking more water whenever you travel, you will have more energy to walk and move around more.

In addition, you will feel full and have less of an urge to eat unhealthy foods or snacks by simply drinking more water.

One tip for making sure you drink enough water whenever you travel to is bring your water bottle with you whenever you travel.

You can simply refill your water bottle at the airport, at the hotel or at a water fountain.

**Sign-up for A Sporting Event**

If you are traveling to another city, state or country, consider signing up for a fun sporting event like a 5K Run, a cycling race, a half marathon or a swimming event.

Whatever kind of fitness you like to do, consider participating in a sporting event because they are fun, they are a great way to explore a city, they will help you to stay focused on your health and fitness goals and you get to travel!!!

**Get Enough Rest (sleep 7-9 hours)**

Traveling is amazing because you get to see and experience many wonderful things.  However, it is important to make sure that you also make time to get enough rest and sleep.

Sometimes when you travel to a different city, state or country you may get super excited and you get this burst of energy that is almost like an adrenaline rush. This burst of energy can keep you going for hours and hours doing many different things.

However, you have to make sure that you are still getting your 7-9 hours of sleep every night in order to continue to have success with your health and fitness goals.

If you stay out late and your sleep suffers then your health and fitness goals will also suffer so remember to get enough rest the next time you travel.

**Do Some Exercise Early in The Morning**

If you have to travel for work, then simply try to go to sleep a little earlier so that you can wake up a little earlier to get a morning workout.

Even if you travel for pleasure, it is a good idea to wake up early and do some exercise immediately upon waking up.

Research shows that doing some form of light exercise upon waking up is a great way to get the body and mind ready for the day.

Your morning workout does not have to be long. You can do a short, intense bodyweight circuit routine in your very own hotel room. You can also simply go for a short 20-minute run or a 30-minute walk.

The point is you want to start your day by being active because later in the day you may get a little lazy and decide not to do any exercise especially if you feel tired.

**Summary**

Maintaining a workout routine or exercise plan while traveling for business or pleasure can help you stay motivated to exercise and stay in shape.

Remember to keep living a health and fitness lifestyle simple. In addition, be strategic and plan ahead before you travel.

By planning ahead, you will be able to live your health and fitness lifestyle wherever you may be.

# Why Use A Kneeling Chair?

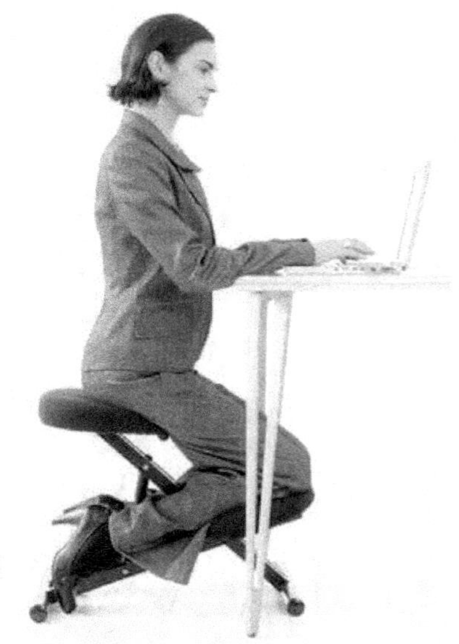

First, what is a kneeling chair?

A kneeling chair is an ergonomic chair that is design to reduce back pain that a person feels when they sit on a regular office chair for long periods of time.

Usually people that have an office desk job or people that work from home tend to suffer from chronic back pain as a result of slouching or hunching over their computers while sitting on a chair.

As time goes by, a person will eventually develop poor posture as a result of improper spinal alignment from sitting hunched over on a computer for long periods of time.

As a result, kneeling chairs were designed for office workers, entrepreneurs that work from home or anyone that wants to use a safer, more comfortable chair.

**Below Are Some of The Benefits of Kneeling Chairs:**

**Improves Posture**

Kneeling chairs are designed in an ergonomic manner which prevents a person from hunching over. As a result, kneeling chairs help prevent any damage to the spine as well as help improve a person's posture.

A kneeling chair positions you to lean forward. While leaning forward, you get all the support that you need to keep your spine aligned properly.

As you begin to use a kneeling chair, you will begin to notice your posture improve even when you are not sitting down.

In addition, when using a kneeling chair, you will almost feel like you are standing but instead you are using your knees and shins to sit upright. So, when you are in an upright position, you will experience less back pain.

Sometimes when a person sits down for a long period of time, that person may experience lower back pain near the tail-bone. As a result of using a kneeling chair, any lower back pain near the tail-bone is completely eliminated as a result of sitting in an upright position.

Because **kneeling chairs help keep the spine in alignment, they are great for reducing back pain.**

**Improves Productivity**
Sitting down on a regular office chair for long periods of time can easily make a person very lazy, tired and unmotivated to do any work.

However, kneeling chairs are designed in a way that prevent any hunching or slumping like you would experience by sitting on a regular office chair.

Because a kneeling chair forces you to lean forward and sit in an upright position, you will be more alert and active then if you were to sit on a regular office chair that allows you to hunch or slouch.

As a result of using a kneeling chair, your energy levels will greatly increase.  In addition, kneeling chairs help fight fatigue as a result of giving you more energy to be more productive and perform better throughout the day.

Because kneeling chairs will increase your energy levels, you are likelier to get up and move around more than if you were to sit in a regular office chair.

Whenever you do get up and more around more, you reduce stiffness in your back from sitting down for long periods of time. In addition, you also reduce chronic back pain when you get up and move around.

Because you will be sitting upright in a more alert manner when using a kneeling chair, you will have the energy to perform better at whatever task you are working on at your desk.

It is also important to state that because you will be sitting in an upright position when using a kneeling chair, you will be engaging your core.

So, when your core is engaged you are actually working out your abdominal muscles and this is great because you are being active as you sit on a kneeling chair.

**Safety**

It is important to state that kneeling chairs safely support the body in an upright position.

Since a kneeling chair safely supports the body in an upright position, you will notice that your posture will also greatly improve as you begin to stand and walk around.

Simply because you are practicing to have good posture while you sit in an upright position you are also training your back and core muscles to develop the habit of walking with good posture as well.

Kneeling chairs are very safe to use because they reduce pressure on a person's spine. In addition, kneeling chairs place the body's weight on the buttocks, shins and knees in a safe and controlled manner.

Kneeling chairs also prevent you from falling over as well as help you to sit in a comfortable more upright position.

A lot of people have reported to feel great as a result of using a kneeling chair. In addition, kneeling chairs are very comfortable to sit on for extended periods of time.

Kneeling chairs can easily help people to work on their computers or laptops without having to suffer from any back pain.

**Summary**

Consider that kneeling chairs are ideal for anyone looking to reduce back pain while improving their posture.

In addition, kneeling chairs are great for office workers, entrepreneurs that work from home or anyone that wants to use a safer, more comfortable chair.

So, if you want to improve your posture, eliminate back pain and sit in a conformable chair, then think about how a kneeling chair can be used at your workplace, home office or some other place.

Also think about how comfortable a kneeling chair will make you feel.

Overall, consistent movement is one of the best ways to decrease lower back pain and improve your posture especially when sitting at a desk for long periods of time.

# The Benefits of a Standing Desk

If you are an office worker or a person that spends a lot of time sitting down surfing the internet you may be doing more harm than good to your body. What you may not know is that sitting down for long periods of time will kill you.

There have been numerous studies showing that sitting for long periods of time is extremely harmful to your health.

For example, sitting down for long periods of time can lead to obesity, neck and back pain as well as cancer, diabetes, a stroke and even heart disease.

However, it is important to state that there is an alternative to sitting down at a traditional desk for long periods of time and that alternative is using a standing desk.

**What Is A Sanding Desk?**

A standing desk is a desk that is designed for a person to use while standing up. A person can use a standing desk to comfortably read, write or do some work on a computer or laptop while standing up.

Here is an interesting question for you:

**Did you know that standing desks were used in the 18<sup>th</sup> and 19<sup>th</sup> century by very wealthy people?**

Here is another interesting question for you:

**Did you know that some famous people that used standing desks were Leonardo Da Vinci, Earnest Hemingway, Benjamin Franklin and Winston Churchill?**

Ok, getting back to standing desks.  There are many kinds of standing desks with all kinds of styles and comforts. However, it is important to find one that is suitable for you.

Below are some of the benefits of using a standing desk:

**A Standing Desk Can Help You to Lose Weight**
Research shows that you burn more calories when using a standing desk then when you sit down and use a traditional desk.

Simply, when you are standing up, your body is using more energy to remain standing versus when you sit down.  When you are sitting down at a traditional desk, all of your weight is being supported by a chair and many times that chair may not even be comfortable.

In addition, standing desks get you moving around more as well as walking around more because you are more motivated to walk or move around then if you sit down at a traditional desk which simply makes the body and mind too comfortable and lazy.

## A Standing Desk Reduces Back Pain

People that sit down and work at a traditional desk for long periods of time have constant complaints of back pain.

Standing desks are known to help a person eliminate back pain as a result of a person being forced to stand up straight instead of being hunched over at a computer screen at a traditional desk.

## A Standing Desk Reduces Heart Disease

Research shows that heart disease is linked to sitting down for long periods of time. However, when a person simply switches to using a standing desk, a person's rate of getting heart disease is quickly reduced as a result of using a standing desk.

Standing up, getting proper circulation throughout the body and moving even for a little bit greatly reduces a person's chance of getting heart disease.

**Standing Desks Reduce Back Pain**

It's a fact…people that sit down for long periods of time while using a traditional desk suffer from sever back pain. However, back pain can tremendously be reduced by using a standing desk.

A standing desk forces you to stand up and have good posture. In addition, your body especially your legs get more circulation when you use a standing desk versus using a traditional desk.

Another benefit of using a standing desk is that it helps to eliminate neck pain from being "hunched" over while sitting working on a computer using a traditional desk.

**A Standing Desk Gives You More Energy**

A standing desk requires you to be more alert because you are standing whereas siting down on a traditional desk can many times make you sleepy and lazy as a result of feeling to comfortable.

This is not to say that standing desks are uncomfortable.  Actually, there are so many different kinds of standing desks that it is easy to find one that is comfortable and suitable for your needs.

But getting back to standing desks giving you more energy, standing desks require you to remain focus on your computer tasks while at the same time preventing you from getting sleepy as a result of having to stand up straight.

In addition, using a standing desk makes you feel less stressed and fatigue especially your lower back and legs because your body especially your lower body gets good circulation from standing up.

A standing desk can also give you the energy to walk around more whether it is in an office environment or at your home office.

Standing desks are also known to improve your mood whereas traditional desks suck your energy and simply make you lazy.

**Standing Desks Prevent Soreness and Cramps**

Standing desks are amazing for avoiding soreness and leg cramps that traditional desks seem to give you.

Standing desks help you to stretch out your legs and provide good circulation throughout the body.

Standing desks also help eliminate aches and pains a person feels around their lower body when sitting for long periods at a time at a traditional desk.

**Standing Desks Burn More Calories**

Standing desks are know to burn more calories than traditional desks because when you are sitting down at a traditional desk, you are doing very little moving.

However, standing desks require you to use more energy and burn more calories as a result of standing upright for extended periods.

**Standing Desks Can Improve Your Productivity Levels**

Standing desks are known to improve productivity levels because unlike sitting down and using a traditional desk, your body is alert and you do not get sleepy and feel tired the same way as if you used a traditional desk.

In addition, a standing desk makes you feel active because you have to stand up straight and you shift your weight from one foot to another.

**Standing Desks Improve Posture**

Sitting down on a traditional desk for long periods of time has been known to affect a person's posture. However, standing desks help improve a person's posture because they require a person to stand up straight instead of hunching over on a chair at a traditional desk.

In addition, standing desks help you to strengthen your core/abs which is another reason why you should use a standing desk.

When you stand up straight while using a standing desk, you are using your core/abs muscles to keep you from hunching over. As a result, you are working out your core/abs while using a standing desk and this helps you to improve your posture.

## Standing Desks Can Help You to Live Longer

Research shows that sitting down for long periods of time reduces a person's life expectancy.

However, when a person stands or adds movement to the body, a person's life expectancy increases.

So, when a person stands for say 20 minutes instead of sitting down, the body is active and working harder to stay upright then when a person simply sits down for long periods of time.

So, what this means is that any kind of small amounts of exercise whether it is standing or walking adds years to your life unlike living a sedentary lifestyle which takes years away from your life.

## Here Are Some Tips for Using a Standing Desk

- If you plan to use a standing desk, make sure you alternate between standing and sitting. For example, sit at your traditional desk for 20 minutes then stand at your standing desk for 20 minutes. Next, take a 10-minute break and begin the cycle again.

- Make sure to use comfortable shoes when using a standing desk.

- Make sure your computer placed on a standing desk is set to your eye level. So, you want to make sure that your computer on your standing desk does not cause you to hunch over or cause any discomfort so adjust your standing desk according to your height.

- Make sure to stand up straight while using a standing desk and make sure to stretch out your legs.

- In addition to using a standing desk for improving your health, you also want to include doing some walking or some other kind of exercises you like to do.

# Conclusion

Thanks for taking the time to read these additional chapters.

I truly hope that these additional chapters regarding improving your overall wellbeing have given you something that you can benefit from when it comes to living a Health and Fitness Lifestyle.

Also, if you enjoyed reading this book, please leave a review on Amazon.

Thanks!